So you've been "Integrated" now what?

*Opportunities For Physicians
Practicing in Managed Care Systems*

BY RICHARD E. THOMPSON, MD

D1080892

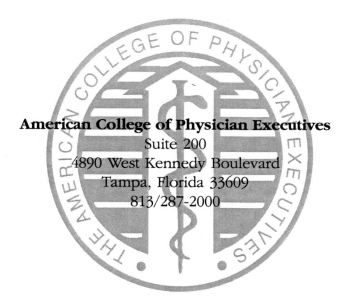

American College of Physician Executives
Suite 200
4890 West Kennedy Boulevard
Tampa, Florida 33609
813/287-2000

ISBN: 0-924674-46-6

Library of Congress Card Number: 96-85458

Printed in the United States by Hillsboro Printing, Tampa, Florida

About the Author

A graduate of Vanderbilt University (AB, 1955), Nashville, Tennessee, and Washington University School of Medicine, St. Louis, Missouri (MD 1959, AOA and cum laude), Richard E. Thompson, MD, is an author and public speaker, well-known in the health care field for his innovative approach to a variety of issues. He has served on the corporate boards of two health care systems.

Dr. Thompson is author of more than 100 published articles and books, including *Keys to Winning Physician Support* (ACPE, 1991), *HealthCare Reform as Social Change* (ACPE, 1993), *The Medical Staff Leader's Practical Guidebook*, 3rd Edition (Opus, 1996), and a humor book, *Things You Will Learn If You Live Long Enough* (Celex/Great Quotations, 1989). He is the developer of "Medical Staff Portfolio," a set of documents governing activities of physicians in medical centers.

Once a practicing pediatrician (1964-70), then Chief of Pediatrics at the Columbus (Georgia) Medical Center and simultaneously Assistant Professor of Pediatrics at Emory University (1970-74), Atlanta, Georgia; Deputy Director of JCAHO's Quality Resource Center (1974-75), Chicago, Illinois; and Vice President of the Illinois Hospital Association (1974-79), Chicago, Illinois, Dr. Thompson has freelanced since 1979.

Dr. Thompson is ACPE's representative to the Professional and Technical Advisory Committee of JCAHO's Accreditation Program for Hospitals/Medical Centers.

How to use this book

Only you know why you bought this book. I can think of three ways you might plan to use it.

First, and best I think, is to read the book and then discuss or debate passages of interest with colleagues and co-workers. Consider using this book to stimulate and focus discussion at a weekend retreat.

Second, you could just skim through or read the book without discussing it with anybody. Why would you do that?

Finally, you could use this and other new books to rotate all the old books off your office shelf and replace them with shinier ones. If you do this, do me a favor, will you? Crack the back of this book and muss up the pages a little. That way, if I ever come to your office, you can show me how critically important this book has been to you in discovering new pathways to personal success.

That will mean a lot to me.

Richard E. Thompson, MD
August 1996

PROLOGUE (IN FOUR SCENES)

Scene 1   **Time:** 1965
            Place: The Doctors' Lounge of Caring
                      Community Hospital

            (Carl Smith, MD, and Ray Miller, MD, are
            relaxing in comfortable chairs.)

Carl: *More coffee?*

Ray: *Not 'til I get to the office.*

Carl: *Seen my gall bladder in 303 yet?*

Ray: *Yep, but I don't think she's a gall bladder. More like an
            ulcer. I ordered all the x-rays and stuff.*

Carl: *She wants to know when she can go home.*

Ray: *Hmmmm. All the studies have got to come back. Plus I'm
            taking a three-day weekend. Tell her ten, twelve days.*

Carl: (Slight pause.) *Seen this morning's paper?*

Ray: *No.*

Carl: *Congress is about to pass that Medicare thing.*

Ray: *The socialized medicine bill?* (Carl nods.)

Carl: *Some day, medical care could be just one more political
            football.*

Scene 2   **Time:** 1980
           Place: The Doctors' Lounge at Caring Community
                Regional Medical Center

(Charles Clark, MD and Ron Milner, MD are going through their mail, which they just took out of their   hospital mailboxes.)

Charles: *Seen my gall bladder in 303?*

Ron: *She can wait. Did you get one of these?*

Charles: *From the hospital lawyer? Yeah. Seems like everybody's included in the suit. I'll swear, the lawyers are in control of everything! (A beat.) What about this one?*

Ron: *The thing from the administrator?*

Charles: *CEO*

Ron: *What the heck's the difference?*

Charles: *None. It's a management thing. Doesn't affect us. Got any denial notices from the PRO?*

Ron: *Sounds like a game of "go fish." (A beat.) Here's another nastygram from Medical Records.* (Tosses it into the waste basket.)

Charles: (Opens another envelope, reads memo.) *Oh, no! They've scheduled the lawyer to speak at the Medical Society the same night as our protest meeting about firing the old Pathology group and hiring one that would work cheaper without asking the Medical Executive Committee first!*

Ron: *That's OK, I'm not going to either meeting. What's the use?*

Scene 3 **Time:** 1995

Place: The Physicians' and Allied Health Care Professionals' Lounge at the West Central Campus location of the Acute Care Medical Services Component of the Vertically and Horizontally Integrated ProfitCare Managed Healthcare System, Caring for More Than 35,000 Covered Lives

(Wayne Smith, MD, and Joseph Langhorn, MD are just entering.)

Wayne: *...So I don't know which one or all of 'em. But some of my most faithful patients are with CareMost. And I gotta be on ProfitCare for the referrals, and CareMore America is putting the squeeze on my partner.*

Joe: *Mildred in my office wants to know, and I think she's right, how she's gonna get all the paperwork done and answer the phone without me hiring another girl or two.*

Wayne: *The primary care guys've got all that taken care of for them with that new Management Service.*

Joe: *Yeah, times have changed. The CEO used to suck up to the cardiologists. Now he plays golf with the family physicians.*

Wayne: (A beat.) *My grandkid wants to be a doctor. Can't talk her out of it.*

Joe: (Lost in his own thoughts.) *I've gotta decide soon. Maybe the easiest thing after all is just let the [censored] buy my practice.*

Scene 4   **Time:** 2005
            Place: The Professional Staff Lounge of MediBest
            Healthcare System

(Carl Smith Jr., MD, and Ray Miller Jr., MD, are seated at computers.)

Carl: *Seen my gall bladder in 303 yet?*

Ray: *Didn't I tell you? She was an ulcer. Sent her home yesterday, with instructions to see you.*

Carl: *Did you get a scan?*

Ray: *Didn't need one.* (A beat. Points to a name on his computer screen.) *When do you want to call in the Ethics committee on this one?*

Carl: *I told Bill about him. He says just go ahead and work with the family, since the Living Will's so clear.*

Ray: *Did you talk to the hospital's attorney?*

Carl: *Who you think did the clear Living Will? Now, it's up to the patient's family and me. Why would we punt back to a lawyer?*

Ray: *Won't the Chief be upset?*

Carl: *Chief of Staff?*

Ray: *No, the CEO.*

Carl: *Not at all. Don't forget, the old guy that was promoted from Chief Finance Officer way back in '81 retired. He'd have been upset. Heck, he wouldn't even get out of bed in the morning without calling the lawyer to ask if his alarm clock went off yet. But the new CEO's cross-trained in both business management and clinical medicine. He understands.*

Ray: *One of those "physician executives?"* (Carl nods.) *I'd never do that.*

Carl: *Well, that's what makes the world go round.*

Contents

PART I. THE PRACTICING PHYSICIAN'S ORGANIZATIONAL ROLE

PART II. THE PRACTICING PHYSICIAN'S CLINICAL ROLE

PART III. THE PRACTICING PHYSICIAN'S ROLE IN
ORGANIZATIONAL FUNCTIONS RELATED TO PATIENT CARE

PART IV. POSITIONING FOR FUTURE DEVELOPMENTS

⊤Chapter 1
THE ROAD IMMEDIATELY AHEAD

[It is not] pre-ordained that medical practitioners will lose control of health care to system integrators and become mere employees of the system.[1]

By the year 2005, practicing physicians will once again be at the center of the U.S. health care system, instead of on the outside looking in. That's because people are beginning to realize what medical care would be like if all the politicians, insurers, executives, attorneys, accountants, and management consultants came to work, but all the doctors stayed at home.

In September 1993, President Bill Clinton announced to the nation (in a joint session of Congress on the night the wrong speech got put on the Teleprompter®) his challenge to Congress to create a uniform health care policy. He asked Congress to enact health care legislation based on six criteria: security, simplicity, savings, quality, choice, and responsibility.[2,3]

This initiative was welcomed by many because of problems (real and perceived) with obtaining dependable, affordable medical care.[4,5,6] But, by 1995, a combination of naive mistakes by President Clinton, self-serving political leadership by Republicans, and effective special interest lobbying had defeated this latest effort[6] to re-form (fundamentally change) U.S. health care policy.

Even as political efforts at reformation sputtered, imaginative health care leaders began a transformation of the U.S. health care system that is only in its first phase and will continue throughout the next decade. (I'd say "into the next millennium," but starting a fresh thousand years has little to do with the real reasons that needed changes are occurring.)

Figure 1. Business Week, October 15, 1984.

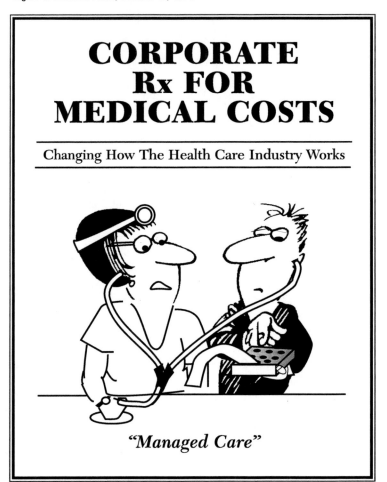

The central feature of this transformation is a change from separatism and overly intense competition to creation of Integrated Health Care Delivery Systems (IHCDSs). These systems will meet all health care needs of served populations, ranging from the pursuit of "wellness," to chiropractic services, to providing dependable critical care on the scariest days of people's "covered lives."

The vision of those transforming the system is that hospitals, medical groups, managed care organizations, nursing homes, clinics, medical instruments and apparatus suppliers, insurance companies—anything you can name having to do with medical care—are merely operational divisions in a much larger organization.

SO YOU'VE BEEN "INTEGRATED": NOW WHAT

The owner of the larger organization may be an insurance company or a provider conglomerate, or a group of investors with no background in medical care settings. There may also be a role for smaller systems confined to a limited geographic area.

The issues of exact organizational structure and ownership are not the subject of this book. The subject of this book is the role of the practicing physician/physician executive team in an integrated system, regardless of the details of organizational structure and ownership.

The first phase of the health care transformation has not been pretty. A rush to integrate, driven by justifiable expectations of investor profit and high executive compensation, has left users of medical care services little better off than in previous years. In fact, this transitional phase in U.S. health care will be recognized by historians as characterized more by legal, financial, and political maneuvering than by genuine interest in providing dependable, affordable medical care.

We are now rapidly moving into the next phase of this transition, characterized by a balanced search for value in health care. This balanced approach means that the success of a health care conglomerate now depends as much on efforts to confirm dependable performance from the view of those needing medical care, as it does on efforts to demonstrate efficient, money-saving management to purchasers and payers.

Enter the practicing physician/physician executive team.

By 2005, because of the need for balanced skills in leading an IHCDS, Boards of Directors will choose senior executives cross-trained in both business management and clinical medicine. There is even today no shortage of "physician executives" to fill this need. Thus, "management" will better understand the needs of practicing physicians committed to delivering dependable medical care to people on the scariest days of their lives.

By 2005, critical life-and-death patient management decisions will once again be the prerogative of physicians, patients, and family members, instead of being involved in a tangle of legalistic fears and technicalities.

By 2005, people will once again remember that, in spite of modern medical miracles and an emphasis on "wellness," the death rate in the United States will always be the same. It's one apiece.

So, by 2005, medicine will once again be a profession, but practiced in a more business-like manner than in the days of "private practice."

Professionally motivated practicing physicians using computers and new advances in clinical technology will enjoy public respect, credibility with the media, political clout, and positions of leadership within Integrated Health Care Delivery Systems (IHCDSs).

Advantages of the Integrated Setting

U.S. physicians, accustomed to a high degree of autonomy, were at first dismayed by the prospect of practicing in a "system." However, an increasing number of practicing physicians now appreciate the advantages to physicians of practicing in an integrated setting.

Example of these advantages include:

Logistical Convenience—The physical setting of an integrated system ordinarily includes physician office space in proximity to a hospital and long-term care facilities, as well as a pharmacy and a "wellness" center. Keep in mind that this is much simpler for patients and family members, too. No more shuffling between specialists, labs, and x-ray/imaging centers scattered randomly around a community. This is only one example of how the integrated approach to delivering health care services can meet the needs of both practitioners and patients.

Simpler Paperwork—The IHCDS may be the insurer paying for the patient's care. Whether or not that is true, billing in the integrated setting will replace the traditional proliferation of disjointed billing efforts by many different organizations.

Fewer Legal Issues—The profit-taking health care model unfortunately invited application of antitrust laws to the health care field and made providers vulnerable under Medicare/Medicaid fraud and abuse statutes. Actually, this attention was justified for a time. The goal of maximizing investor profit generated a number of arrangements between physicians and health care organizations that made old-time "fee-splitting" look like child's play.

Integration of medical services changes that scenario. In the eyes of the law, cross-referrals between physicians within a single system (including referrals for laboratory, x-ray, and imaging studies) are seen as motivated by patient need, not ploys to raise physician income. In addition, better public-provider relations in a system clearly designed to meet the needs of the public should lead to reducing the number of nuisance malpractice suits against physicians and hospitals.

Good Patient Care—Some physicians believe that people using medical care services will not like the integrated approach.

Au contraire.

Pretend you are the patient. Care should be available, good, and affordable. Physician-guided cross-referrals should decrease the possibility of inadvertent selection by patients of a marginally performing physician.

Perhaps above all, continuity of care for each patient and family is best ensured by an integrated approach. The security thus achieved for people with chronic medical problems should pay dividends to physicians by enhancing (one could say restoring) the physician's public image as a concerned professional.

So, successful practicing physicians will not dwell on what might be lost in the brave new world of integrated systems. (Actually, some of the "advantages" of freestanding private practice were illusory at best.) Instead, the successful practicing physician will focus on, and add to, the list of advantages to be gained by practicing in a system, with a carefully chosen staff of qualified and committed practitioners available for consultation and coverage, with management support that frees the physician to concentrate on medical practice, and with renewed public confidence in physicians that can translate into greater political support as well.

A Roadmap

The immediate road ahead is marked by confusing and sometimes contradictory road signs. A safe journey depends on carefully distinguishing between four similar-sounding concepts. These are managed competition, managed care system, integrated health care delivery system (IHCDS), and managed care.

Managed competition is a market-controlled, profit-taking system controlling the flow of health care dollars. It is not new, having started as part of the Reagan administration's "trickle down economics" policies. In this profit-taking system, the primary goal of health care executives is to maximize profit for investors.

In the Great Health Care Reform Debate of 1993-94, which focused only on the question of how U.S. health care should be financed, this profit-taking model was pitted against the "single-payer" model for

Figure 2. St. Pete Times, March 27, 1994. Universal Press Syndicate.

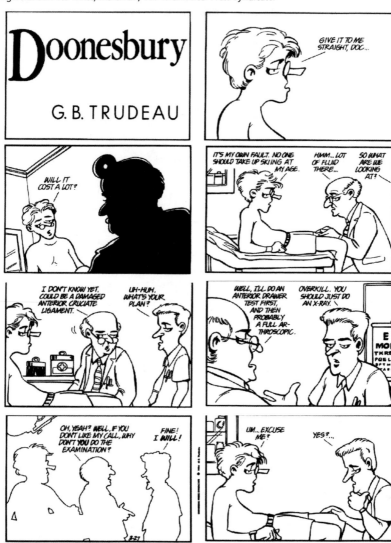

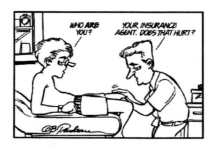

SO YOU'VE BEEN "INTEGRATED": NOW WHAT

financing health care. The single-payer model was championed by those who could envision a simpler system with lower administrative costs. The profit-taking managed competition model was championed by those benefiting from such a model, such as insurance companies, health care executives, and Wall Street financiers.

The biggest issue in this debate was trust. The primary objection to the single-payer model was distrust of big government. The primary objection to the managed competition model was distrust of big business.

Naturally, the profit-taking model won, because the seduction of the profit-taking model is almost impossible to resist. However, an increasing number of knowledgeable people fear that the profit-taking model might eventually lead to unpredicted consequences. For example, draining away of health care dollars into investor profit, combined with heavy debts resulting from leveraging during the acquisition phase of this transition, might lead to inadequate maintenance and replacement of medical equipment. The result could be dilapidated health care facilities without updated capabilities.

The profit-taking, managed competition model for financing health care, unique in the world, was conceived in a society driven by the notion that the primary goal of all endeavors, including those once considered professions, is investor profit. Features of managed competition increasingly realized by a frustrated public include distracting antitrust issues, concern about dependability of services if the primary goal is profit ("cut the losers, regardless of people's needs"), and the use of health care dollars to pay for trappings of the profit-taking model, including marketing costs, high executive salaries, and investor profit. It is likely that managed competition is a short-lived fad.

A **managed care system** is an amalgam of providers created to take advantage of the profit-taking health care model. An integrated delivery system can exist without the assumption that the goal of the system is investor profit.

An **integrated health care delivery system (IHCDS)** is an amalgam of health care providers whose goal is to provide a full range of medical care services throughout the lives of beneficiaries or members of the integrated system. This concept favors the interests of people needing medical care of all kinds and need not injure the interests of providers. This idea is here to stay.

Managed care is a term used by some to refer to the profit-taking, managed competition, market-driven model of financing U.S. health care. Others use this term in an individual patient context. Physicians have always talked about "managing the patient." Since the advent of managed competition, managed care in the context of diagnosing and treating an individual patient has focused on cutting costs. (See figures 1-1 and 1-2, pages 00 and 00.)

However, in the context of treating patients in an IHCDS without so much focus on the profit motive, managed care using practice guidelines and clinical pathways is relevant to achievement of good patient results as well as to cost concerns. In tailoring practice guidelines to the unique features of each patient, overutilization will be avoided, keeping patient discomfort to a minimum as well as holding down costs.

In the sense of using reasonable practice guidelines as a template for designing a care plan for each individual patient, managed care is definitely a positive part of practicing in an IHCDS. (See Chapter 7.)

References

1.   The Atlanta Consulting Group. *America's Healthcare: The Big Squeeze.* La Jolla, Calif.: The Governance Institute, 1996, , p. 2.

2.   Clinton, B. "The Clinton Health Care Plan." *New England Journal of Medicine* 327(11):804-6, Sept. 10, 1992.
3.   President Bill Clinton. Address to Joint Session of Congress. Sept. 22, 1993.

4.   Shortell, S., and McNerney, W. "Criteria and Guidelines for Reforming the U.S. Health Care System." *New England Journal of Medicine* 322(7):463-6, Feb. 15, 1990.

5.   Blendon, R., and others. "Satisfaction With Health Systems in 10 Nations." *Health Affairs* 9(3):185-92, Summer 1990.

6.   Thompson, R. *Health Care Reform as Social Change.* Tampa, Fla.: American College of Physician Executives, 1993.

Chapter 2

ORGANIZATIONAL ROLES AVAILABLE TO PHYSICIANS

The doctor whose personal authority in the Nineteenth Century rested on his imposing character and relations with patients was in a fundamentally different situation from the doctor in the Twentieth Century whose authority depends on holding the necessary credentials and institutional affiliations.[1]

The first step toward living with integration is pausing to consider a short list of the only roles available in any organization and consciously choosing one (or two, or three) roles to play.

This fact is not news to some physicians, who have learned something about how organizations work in pre-med courses or as a result of practical work experience. However, the practicing physician's basic training (medical school and residency) does little to help him or her adapt to an organizational setting. In fact, the "subtle curriculum" of medical school and residency training suggests that it is the organization that should adapt to the physician. (You've heard how many doctors it takes to screw in a light bulb? Only one. He stands on a ladder holding the light bulb while the whole world revolves around him.)

"It takes the whole first year of law school," an attorney friend told me, "just to learn to think like a lawyer. And once you do, it's hard to think any other way." The same is true of medical training. It takes the whole first year of medical school just to learn to think like a practicing physician. That process is far removed from thinking about oneself as part of an organization. In fact, part of learning to think like a practicing doctor is learning to isolate oneself from others, and from the way others think.

In the anatomy lab, I must not think of this cadaver as a person. I must become detached and totally objective. (There is very little difference between the words "clinical" and "cynical.")

I must think quickly and act decisively and independently. I must pay little attention to those who urge me to gather more complete information before acting. For one thing, information is unreliable. (Physicians evaluate the validity of a history from the patient; "70 percent reliable" is a really good score for people being asked to recall events in an illness.)

In addition, my patient's best interests depend on my willingness to begin immediate treatment without having all test results back yet.

I must never be guilty of an incomplete "work-up." I must order every test available on my patient so the attending physician won't embarrass me on "rounds" by pointing out a diagnostic test that I failed to order.

And, of course, I must never be guilty of withholding any available diagnostic or treatment modality from any patient. I must do "everything possible," with emphasis on "everything." I must resist the notions of irreversible medical conditions and death. To a good doctor, intractable illness and death are defeats.

Whether I'm a "thinking doctor" (e.g., internist) or a "cutting doctor" (e.g., surgeon), my patient's life and health depend on my exhibiting these behaviors at all times and standing firm against those who might try to persuade me otherwise.

This is a difficult responsibility. Of course, I'm encouraged by the fact that society obviously recognizes the special nature of my authority and the strain on me at all times. For example, I'm always excused from jury duty, no questions asked. After all, I'm a doctor.

No wonder the fledgling MD or DO emerges from medical school believing that there is only one role for all doctors. That role is Unquestioned Captain of the Ship. Of course, that must mean Captain of any and all ships the MD or DO chooses to sail on.

What a shock it is, then, to discover that the MD or DO who wishes to be successful in an integrated setting must choose one (or two, or three) specific organizational roles to play. And what a shock to discover even further that even practicing physicians are subject to performance evaluation. By superiors!

But after the initial shock wears off, the MD or the DO realizes two things. First, this business of choosing a role really isn't new to me. For example, I wasn't born a doctor. I could have chosen to be a real estate agent or a fishing guide. I'm a doctor because I chose that role in life. Then I chose a role within the medical profession. I could've been a primary care "gatekeeper" or a tertiary care specialist such as a cardiac surgeon instead of a secondary care specialist such as an obstetrician/gynecologist. Come to think of it, whatever my schedule is today and this week and this month, it reflects my own choice of roles from among many available to well-educated and thinking people in this great country. Hmmmmm.

Second, there are more roles available than I knew there were. If more than one role interests me, why couldn't I explore the possibility of simultaneously playing two or three? Hmmmmm. Not so bad, after all.

Available Roles

To understand the concept of "organizational roles," think about making a movie. The desired result of movie-making is a good movie that generates a profit for investors. That result can be achieved only by cooperative efforts of several people. Each person on the movie-making team must accomplish a given task. For example, some (actors) will play on-screen roles. While the on-screen actors are the most visible part of a movie, the contribution of others is equally critical. You know this from watching the overly long Oscar Night awards show on TV every year. Best Screenplay, Best Lighting, Best Adapted Screenplay with Original Music, Best Sound Effects, etc. The list seems endless.

But the list is not endless. Only certain roles are available on the movie-making team. One can choose "Writer." (Leave it to a writer to remind you that good on-screen performances aren't possible unless the writer gives the actor a character to develop.) One might choose director, or wardrobe supervisor. Given enough money, one could be the movie's producer.

By the way, given a choice between producer and any other team role, always choose producer. Others may take pride in knowing the movie cannot be made without them. But others (even the director) must expect occasional frustration when they disagree with a decision made by the producer, whose authority prevails.

In an integrated health care delivery setting, the desired result is providing dependable medical services of all kinds. (Whether or not investor profit should be included as a desirable result in integrated health care systems is a question that will be up in the air for several more years.) The desired result of the IHCDS's efforts can only be achieved by individuals who choose specific roles. Everybody contributes to the failure or the success of the IHCDS.

The short list of roles available to MDs and DOs in integrated systems include owner, member of the board of directors, executive (CEO or vice president of something), clinical leader/manager (such as director of ob/gyn services), or practicing physician (the front-line worker role).

If you go for practicing physician, take pride in knowing that the desired result of good medical care probably depends on you more than on anyone else in this scenario. But also understand that you must expect occasional frustration when you disagree with a decision made by the CEO and board of directors, whose authority prevails.

A Short Summary of Organizational Roles

The **owners** of an enterprise (including investors) provide capital, call the shots, and expect profits.

The members of the **board of directors** are owner representatives and are expected to establish policies governing activities of the enterprise. The board of an IHCDS is responsible, both legally and morally, for the dependability of medical care provided, as well as for the financial stability of the IHCDS.

The **CEO** (chief executive officer or president) of an enterprise is selected by the board of directors to exercise the board's authority in managing day-to-day activities of the enterprise.

Several **vice presidents of something** are selected by the CEO, so that the CEO can get home to his or her family by 11 pm on weekdays and by early afternoon on Saturday and Sunday. In an IHCDS, the vice president of medical affairs is a senior executive responsible to the CEO and the board for (among other things) performance of practicing physicians in various components of the system.

Directors/managers (such as the human resources director, the director of information services, the director of ob/gyn services, etc.) are selected by the relevant vice president, with approval of the CEO and board. (In today's multilayered IHCDS, a long series of approval steps can slow effective decision making and action taking almost as much as did the series of committee approval steps in the old hospital organized medical staff.)

In most modern-day organizations, the director/manager level is the first level at which there is genuine understanding of day-to-day, person-by-person problems and activities related to serving customers, clients, residents, members, beneficiaries, or patients.

The **practicing physician** role in the IHCDS might be termed the "worker" role in other enterprises. However, in most other enterprises, the "work force" includes individuals with various levels of formal education and some without the internal motivation inherent in people who have chosen to enter professions such as teaching and medicine.

To avoid internal strife and deep depression among practicing physicians, it's best for management-trained executives to understand that physicians don't like to be referred to as a "work force."

Of course, in any organization, it is the workers dealing firsthand with individual consumers (or patients, or clients, or residents—whatever is relevant to the reader) who have the best technical skills, the best knowledge of suitable product design, the best ideas for employee benefits, and the best feel for whether or not "users of the product" are truly pleased with the efforts of the enterprise. This fact was rediscovered in the United States around 1990, when companies were urged to use "continuous quality improvement" techniques to get input from workers.[2] And to pay attention to the input!

Go Ahead, Wear Two Hats

Some organizational roles are often combined. It's not unusual for the director of a movie also to be the producer, or for a part owner of an IHCDS also to be on the board of directors.

But some organizational roles are seldom combined. Show me movie credits listing one person as both star actor and gaffer, or an annual report from an IHCDS with an elegant portrait photograph of a vice president of medical affairs who is also still a practicing physician.

In IHCDSs, some roles are combined by definition. The clinical director of ob/gyn services absolutely must be an ob/gyn specialist, and he or she probably will be combining the roles of clinical director and practicing physician.

Keys to Combining Organizational Roles

Here are some tips for MDs or DOs who wish to combine "practicing physician" with some other organizational role:

- **Don't try to combine "practicing physician" with "vice president of something."** These are both full-time positions. A vice president who must leave a meeting to tend to a patient with a medical emergency just when a critical decision is about to be made is not a fully participating vice president. And a practicing physician who must leave care of his patients to others because, as vice president, he is in a series of meetings all day may be doing a disservice to people by trying to carry a patient load.

- **Prepare yourself well for all roles you choose to play.** Clinical skill (diagnosing and treating patients) is one thing. Organizational skill (analyzing information, motivating people) is another. If you're a practicing physician accepting an organizational leadership role for the first time, expect to give time to learning some new skills.

- **Check with your family.** The practicing physician who agreed to be the unpaid chief of ob/gyn in the good old days was only expected to show up once a month and run a meeting. Today's paid director of ob/gyn services in the IHCDS or one of its components is expected to be available in a timely manner, all the time. Even with an assistant director (or vice chief, if you still prefer the old terminology) available, clinical director is a time-consuming job. Don't let anyone tell you otherwise.

- **Don't accept an organizational position for obstructive reasons.** That is, don't agree to take some organizational decision-making role just to keep someone else from holding the position (out of the fear that the person in that position might make decisions interfering with your practice). That kind of behavior isn't good for the organization. And such self-serving behavior will also eventually prove self-defeating.

- **Don't confuse organizational leadership roles with other kinds of physician leader roles.** For example, leadership in the state or county medical society or the American Medical Association is *political* leadership. Political leaders are position-takers. Physician leaders in organized medicine must, by definition, focus primarily on the needs of physicians.

  In contrast, leadership in the IHCDS is *organizational* leadership. Organizational leaders are problem-solvers. Physician leaders in the IHCDS must focus simultaneously on the needs of the public, on preserving the good public image and fiscal integrity of the IHCDS, and on the needs of the practicing physicians on whom the IHCDS and its beneficiaries depend.

- **Wear the right hat at the right time.** Finally, if you choose to wear more than one hat, be absolutely sure you know when to wear which hat. For example, if you are both a practicing physician and director of ob/gyn services, know when your concern for your patient (practicing physician hat) must give way to concern for patients of all ob/gyn specialists (director of ob/gyn services hat).

Facilitating the Choice of Organizational Roles

Management-trained executives in IHCDSs can make it easier for physicians to understand and choose from available roles. To make the physician's task of choosing a role easier:

- Provide information about available roles, such as the information in this chapter, to practicing physicians on the medical roster of the IHCDS.

- Offer to meet with physicians individually to find out what their questions and concerns are.

- Be up front. If a role that a physician wants to choose is not available, or is filled, say so.

- Above all, show great respect for and establish rewards for MDs and DOs who choose the practicing physician role. It seems necessary to say this, because in recent years health care executives have primarily rewarded entrepreneurial leaders and physicians who wished to become managers or physician executives.

References

1. Starr, P. *The Social Transformation of American Medicine.* New York, N.Y.: Basic Books, 1982, p. 21.

2. Walton, M. *The Deming Management Method.* New York, N.Y.: Dodd, Mead, and Company, 1986.

H Chapter 3
HOW TO CHOOSE THE ORGANIZATIONAL ROLE THAT'S RIGHT FOR YOU

Life's Four Biggest Questions

Who am I?
Why am I here?
Where am I going?
Where are the cookies?

—*Anonymous*

In the integrated health care system, as in most organizations, roles are not chosen. They are assigned. So in one way, a more honest title for this chapter would be, "Which Role Should I Apply for, Hoping to Be Among the Chosen for That Role?"

The First Step: Get to Know Yourself Better

Positioning yourself to be chosen for a role you really want to play starts with taking time to know yourself better. In this self-examination, don't talk yourself into any illusions. Who are you, really? Where are you, in terms of age, life-style, unfulfilled ambitions, family life? Where would you really like to be? OK, Hawaii is good, but also, what are your goals for the rest of your life? What makes you really want to get up in the morning? That is, what kinds of activities do you really get enthusiastic about? OK, golf is good, but what kinds of work activities? Do you enjoy working as a loner or as part of a group? What are your financial goals for yourself and your family, in terms of both annual income and eventual net worth?

I'm not just writing to see myself write. I really want you take a little introspective time for yourself. I know I'm asking a lot here. Meaningful self-examination is not an activity at which physicians are known to excel. I'm a doctor; who has time to think? And who needs it, anyway? Didn't I tell you? I know who I am. I'm a doctor.

Not good enough. Throughout medical school and residency training, the fledgling physician is focused entirely on an intense, grueling effort to learn all about the status, maintenance, and repair of the human body and mind. But that's somebody else's body and mind we're learning about. We hardly ever internalize what we're learning. (Except Dave Stone, in my medical school class. Stony had a new disease every time we switched clinical rotations. During our six weeks on thoracic surgery, he kept going around percussing his own chest, asking, "Wonder how my tumor's coming?" During our six weeks on ob/gyn, Stony thought he had the first case of pre-eclampsia in a nonpregnant male.)

To paraphrase the luxury car ads: Spend some time thinking about yourself. You deserve it. Here are some pointers about specific steps to take. In three or four contemplative sessions of no more than one hour each, do the following (if you can't make yourself set aside even that much time for this exercise, you know something about yourself already):

● Sit down with pencil and paper, or at your word processor if that's how you think best,

● Brainstorm. That means don't judge your thoughts as they come to you. If the thought is in you, let it come all the way to the surface and write it down. Really let your mind "free-wheel." That is, don't let either preconceived notions or negative thoughts ("Oh, I could never do that") into your mind right now. Here's a list of questions to get you started:

   ▸ Why did I go to medical school?

   ▸ What do I like best about being an MD or a DO?

   ▸ What do I like least about being an MD or a DO?

   ▸ What is (are) my professional goal(s)?

   ▸ What is (are) my personal goal(s)?

   ▸ What is (are) my financial goal(s)?

   ▸ What are my personal strengths?

   ▸ What are my personal weaknesses?

   ▸ Would my family, colleagues, and co-workers agree with the answers to the last two questions? (If not, maybe I better go back and be a little more honest with myself, not talking myself into any illusions.)

   ▸ What skills do I have?

- What skills would I most like to develop?

- How much tolerance for authority do I have? That is, can I accept and follow rules, if they're reasonable rules, even if I have no part in mandating the rule?

- Who's my favorite doctor acquaintance? Why? Do I want to be like him or her? Why or why not?

- Who's a doctor acquaintance I really hate to see coming?

- Do I enjoy "the group process," being active in organized groups such as civic clubs, church, or schools? Or do I find meetings, group discussions, and "organizational decision-making" a bore, or even unnecessary?

- Add your own thought-starting questions to this list.

Expect to be tired after each contemplative session. But expect it to be a good tired. You'll enjoy the exercise more as you become more comfortable with the fact that inside your doctor mind and body is a real person.

This self-inspection really doesn't have to go on for days and days. Stop whenever you feel you're to "maximum benefit achieved."

If you have a family, the exercise should include one "Family Council" session of 30 minutes or an hour. Explain that you're trying to define yourself better. When the wisecracks and laughing have died down, ask each family member to suggest what they think your strengths and weaknesses are, and what their goals are.

Finally, photocopy all the notes you've taken. Keep one copy out where you can read over the notes once in awhile. Put the original notes in a manila folder, and put the folder away in a safe but accessible place. (Playwrights do this. They call this folder of notes about themselves their "Credo." The good ones refer to their "Credo" frequently while writing a play, to make their characters consistent and believable and their plots interesting.)

Now, Speak Up!

He who tooteth not his own horn, the same shall not be tooted.— Shakespeare.

Don't sit around hoping that all the leaders in your integrated system will divine that you've discovered what you most enjoy doing, and what you're best at. Ask for a one-hour conference with the vice president of medical affairs or with the chief operating officer in charge of stuff, or whoever in this multilayered, multi-acronymed system is in charge of assigning roles to physicians.

Now, SELL YOURSELF.

Example 1: "Charlie" (Charlie is the CEO or a vice president), "the other cardiac surgeons and I enjoy what we do best, and we don't understand why you don't understand what that is. We are clinical thinkers and surgical technicians. We are part physiologist, part engineer, and part psychologist who spend 20 hours a day, even though there are six of us, making people's hearts work a few years longer.

What we don't do, Charlie, is organizations. We don't belong to the PTA, the Rotary Club, or Ducks Unlimited. Understand what I'm telling you here? Don't be putting us on a whole bunch of committees. We hate committees. Leave us alone in our world. You'll be glad you did."

Example 2: "Charlie, I've been a primary care physician here now for three years. I think I could help you improve some of the clinical and clerical systems we're having to deal with. If you and the other executives are ever sitting around trying to identify some clinicians who would be interested in developing some organizational skills and helping run things around here, just keep me in mind, OK?"

OR

"Charlie, _____

_____

_____

_____

_____."

That's you. Fill in the blanks.

In organizational jargon, here's the bottom line. I can't tell you how to succeed in an integrated system. But I can tell you how to fail. Failure is almost ensured if you accept a role that requires that you be something other than yourself.

A Word to the Wise

After you develop your "Credo," you will know whether you are Dr. Yesterday, Dr. Today, or Dr. Tomorrow. Frankly, Dr. Tomorrow has the best chance of reaping success as a practicing physician in an IHCDS.

Dr. Yesterday would have bristled at the suggestion that a practicing physician should have to further define him- or herself and engage in cooperative effort. I can hear Dr. Yesterday even yet. "A doctor is a doctor is a doctor. These are God's hands. Out of my way. My patient needs me. Everybody else's needs be damned."

The idea that a physician should stoop to letting a "superior" know about personal and professional strengths runs counter to Dr. Yesterday's continued expectation that medical doctors should be granted total autonomy. After all, the only evaluation of performance worth its salt is called "peer review," meaning that only other doctors need to know doctors' strengths and weaknesses. And, of course, that only applies to strengths and weaknesses in terms of applying clinical knowledge and skills to individual patient care encounters. Whatever else makes Dr. Yesterday tick, he or she figures, is nobody else's business.

Dr. Today is somewhat more accepting of the real world. Dr. Today accepts the notion that he or she has to get hired by, or get a contract with, some organization. But Dr. Today doesn't like it. And this doctor mistrusts the integrated system's executive staff and board, even though many of them have MD or DO degrees. After all, they aren't real doctors, having "gone over to the other side." But what choice does Dr. Today have? So he or she signs on, without enthusiasm.

In contrast, Dr. Tomorrow blends acceptance of reality with a vision of the future. For starters, Dr. Tomorrow wouldn't dream of practicing any other way except in an integrated system. He or she welcomes the organizational support, such as office management, that allows him or her to focus on practicing medicine. This doctor welcomes and enjoys the professional satisfaction of working with a carefully selected group of colleagues whose clinical skills, availability, and enjoyment of clinical medicine are a near-match for his or her own. Dr. Tomorrow takes full advantage of opportunities offered to provide input to management about the realities of clinical practice and is gratified when he or she can see that he or she has influenced business decisions made by the system, based on that understanding.

Finally, Dr. Tomorrow is happy with his or her pay and life-style. He or she enjoys the financial security of a salary that is among the top 10 percent across all businesses and professions, nationwide, and the practice coverage to pursue recreational interests and spend time with the family.

Don't believe me? Check it out. Here's how. Mark your computer calendar for January 1, 2005. No, make that January 3, 2005. January 1 that year is a Saturday. Buy a doctor a cup of coffee. Any doctor. Ask the doctor how he or she likes the following new idea for entering the practice of medicine. The fledgling practicing physician will go out and make a decision on which other physicians (if any) to practice with, find suitable office space, hire personnel, set up patient record and bookkeeping systems, buy the medical equipment necessary to practice his or her chosen specialty, borrow heavily, take time to build a practice, and hardly ever see his or her family, at least until he or she can afford to "take in a partner."

The doctor in 2005 will tell you that you're crazy, not very imaginative, or both. Why would a doctor, or a group of doctors, want to invite those hassles? Why would they think they can set themselves up a better practice than has been set up by the physician executives and physician managers in this integrated system? Why wouldn't any physician want the ready availability of specialty consultation? Oh, sure, when things were all screwed up in the 1990s and the "gatekeeper" concept got blown out of proportion by people who made it a stiff, absolute, extra, expensive layer of the patient care process, that was different. But now? Why would anyone think it's a good idea to have a medical practice office anywhere other than in or attached to a hospital building? Most amazing of all, why would anyone try to build a practice alone? Especially when physicians' salaries in the integrated system match or exceed those of physicians who chose to train themselves to be system CEOs.

Make no mistake about it. Dr. Tomorrow is as frustrated as anyone with the layers of management bureaucracy that are currently the focus in "managed care settings" (integrated delivery systems). But Dr. Tomorrow has a positive vision of the integrated system of the not-too-distant future, in which choosing a role is not synonymous with organizational distractions. Rather, choosing a role is synonymous with being able to focus on practicing the best darned medicine the physician knows how to practice.

Best of all, Dr. Tomorrow isn't just sitting around waiting for the vision of tomorrow to come true like a dream. *Au contraire.* Dr. Tomorrow has positioned him- or herself to be in the thick of turning today's out-of-control, profit-taking interpretation of an integrated system into tomorrow's integrated delivery system, profitable because the focus is on patient care.

R Chapter 4
REWARDING THE DOCTOR WHO CHOOSES THE PRACTICING PHYSICIAN ROLE

Caring for patients continues to be the nucleus of activity around which all health care organization functions revolve.[1]

Doctor, take a break. I want to talk to management for a chapter, on your behalf.

Sometimes it seems to practicing physicians that health care executives and boards of directors want every physician to become an executive or a manager. That can't be true. Winning executives and board members understand that only doctors (working with other clinically trained health care professionals who are also essential) can deliver the company's product.

Here are some thoughts about how to show doctors who choose the role of practicing physician that executives and managers appreciate their indispensable contribution to the success of the integrated system.

Executive Rewards versus Physician Rewards

The board should ensure that the reward system for practicing physicians is equivalent, in value, to the reward system for senior executive staff. But the reward system for practicing physicians is a different package, because physician rewards should not be based on what is important to executives. Physician rewards should be based on what is important to practicing physicians. A reward system for practicing physicians established on the basis of what is important to executives will not yield organizational benefits such as careful performance and low personnel turnover.

Rewarding today's business executives is simple. Not easy, maybe, because it's costly. But figuring out how to reward business executives is simpler than figuring out how to reward physicians.

In today's executive-driven world, the senior executive's preferred reward is money, in some form or another. To today's senior executives in all American business, life is simple. Maximize profits to maximize personal wealth of investors, and the investors, through the board of directors, will in turn maximize the executive's personal wealth. (Unfortunately, this is no secret anymore. Excessive executive compensation is a growing issue in this country.)

Over the years, executives have made the mistake of setting up physician reward systems that assume that the same thing is true of doctors. But "rewarding physicians" is not just a euphemism for paying doctors more money.

Now, don't misunderstand the point. Money certainly is one part of a physician's reward system. Send me a check, and I'll keep it. But the reality, believe it or not, is that money is not the only motivation, or even the main driving motivation, of many practitioners who exhibit the characteristics of a sought-after practicing physician (see Chapter 5). Indeed, believe it or not, money is third or fourth or fifth on the list of rewards desired by many physicians. (Frankly, this isn't to say that physicians are all that beneficent. If you've got a few hundred thousand invested on interest and in real estate, it's not so hard to be altruistic.)

The best way to find out what's important to your practicing physicians (in addition to money) is, ASK your practicing physicians! Here are some things that practicing physicians say are really important to them[2,3]:

- Gain practicing physician input before executives and the board make decisions affecting space, staff, and equipment needed to provide dependable medical care.

- Respect clinicians. Some practicing physicians wonder why some health care executives seem to respect only doctors who want to become physician executives and managers.

- Provide relevant, locally presented, continuing medical education opportunities.

- When the purpose of a meeting is announced as "to obtain physician input," physicians say, "let us talk and listen to us," rather than turning the occasion into a presentation of a program or an activity that the executive management staff has already decided it wants to implement but that requires "physician support."

- Offer an excellent, committed staff of nurses and clinical technicians. Streamline "quality improvement" and other functions in which practicing physicians are expected to participate. Require less practicing physician time in administrative-activity meetings.

- "We are always being told what the board of directors needs us to do. Let us hear, at least occasionally, that the CEO went to bat for the practicing physician staff and their patient care responsibilities at a board of directors meeting."
- Pay liability (malpractice) insurance premiums.
- Have adequate reserve funds to maintain and upgrade capital equipment, such as imaging machines and intensive care monitors.
- Keep promises. If something can't be done, don't promise it will be done. Rather, say up front that it can't be done, and say why.

Here are some additional details regarding these thoughts on rewarding physicians.

Pay Money

Pay scales must reward front-line practicing physicians as much as they reward the executive staff and the management support staff. Fringe benefits must be generous and flexible, so that immediate and long-range financial security are ensured, as long as the practicing physician's performance record is good. (See Chapter 9.)

Pay Respect

A key component of the "work force" in the health care business is a staff of self-motivated doctors and nurses. Respect for a person's professionalism and personal integrity is important to many who chose medicine as their lifetime occupation.

Participation in Organizational Decision Making

To a business-trained executive, the primary concern is profit. But a clinically trained physician may be most concerned with the issue of control. That means both control of factors necessary to provide dependable medical care and control of one's own agenda in the context of organizational affairs.

Mechanisms must be in place to ensure that, within reason, practicing physicians are participants in organizational decisions affecting their practice activities. (See Chapter 10.) One advantage of such mechanisms is avoidance of the unnecessary conflict generated when an individual or a group is angered more by lack of participation in a decision than by the decision itself.

Note: As more and more individuals with clinical training (doctors, nurses) assume senior executive positions in management, the issues of lack of respect and inadequate participation in organizational decisions will be less troublesome to practicing physicians than in the past.

CME Opportunities

The organization should provide paid opportunities for physicians to attend conferences and participate in hands-on clinical training sessions relevant to physicians' areas of practice.

Teaching Opportunities

The system's practicing physicians should be asked to participate in in-service education and orientation of nurses and other clinical personnel and in community education programs and should be encouraged to serve as clinical faculty and preceptors for medical students and medical residents in training.

In addition to viewing these opportunities as physician "perks," system management should appreciate the economic value to the IHCDS of this physician visibility, rather than worrying that the physician's teaching time is "not revenue-producing." (See Chapter 11.)

The Question of Bonuses and Incentives Tied to Utilization

Physician bonuses and incentives tied to decreased utilization, such as ordering fewer diagnostic tests, are a terrible idea. If the profit-taking U.S. health care model is ever replaced by a government-controlled single-payer model, history may record that public demand for that change began with concern that clinical decisions became contaminated by personal profit interests.

Physician bonuses that tempt physicians to skimp on providing medical services to an individual will be short-lived in IHCDSs where practicing physicians truly participate in organizational decision making. (This is only one example of how individuals cross-trained in both management and clinical medicine can help executives trained only in finance and business avoid critical mistakes in judgment.)

Organizational Status

True or False? The traditional model of the "organized medical staff" in hospitals is obsolete, and it is counter productive to bring this model forward into today's managed care settings. *(Answer: True.)*

True or False? The relationship of most practicing physicians to the organization in which they practice is now (or soon will be) either through a contractual agreement or employment. *(Answer: True.)*

True or False? The two previous true statements add up to the conclusion that the place of the practicing physician in an integrated health care system is now no more than "labor" in a traditional "labor vs. management" adversarial sense. *(Answer: Totally, absolutely, undeniably, and unequivocally false!)*

The term "medical staff" must no longer be considered synonymous with the traditional two-bylaws, committee-rich, bulky, and slow-moving "organized medical staff" still found in many U.S. hospitals. But, at the same time, the unique nature of a staff of medical professionals, with its collegial nature and useful insights, must not be completely lost, even amidst the reality of contract and employment relationships that will now be the mechanisms through which most physicians are bound to the IHCDS.

From Medical Staff to Professional Staff

OK, doctor, now I'm talking to you again. This is still about organizational status; it's about sharing your organizational status with other clinically trained health care professionals.

Practicing physicians should expect that some IHCDSs may prefer the concept of "professional staff" to the concept of "medical staff." That is, clinically trained individuals, including physicians, nurses, and technicians, might become the "professional staff" of an IHCDS, in contrast to the "executive and management staff" of the IHCDS.

Traditional-thinking practicing physicians may find such a suggestion abhorrent. Especially those politically active physicians who, in the past few years, have chosen to use the "organized medical staff" and its "bylaws" as a bunker from which to wage a last-ditch battle against change.

However, contemporary-thinking physicians will view the broader emphasis as an advantage. For one thing, this alignment reflects a balanced search for value in health care, with as much priority given by management to professional issues as to financial issues.

In addition, over time, physicians will come to understand that having a total professional staff is a competitive advantage. It is hard to imagine a group of physicians who would argue that, in today's world, a group of physicians could compete effectively without including almost all major specialties and subspecialties in the group. How, then, could an IHCDS and its professional staff claim to provide a full range of medical services to an increasingly aging and arthritic population without chiropractic physicians and perhaps even an acupuncturist or two?

Where the line is drawn will be decided in joint discussions among the IHCDS's physician leaders, board, and executive stafff. The point here is that practicing MDs and DOs should expect IHCDS management to provide all needed health care professionals, even those with limited licenses, their share of rewards and respect.

References

1. *Comprehensive Accreditation Manual for Hospitals.* "Introduction to MS.6." Oak Brook, Ill.: Joint Commission on Accreditation of Healthcare Organizations, 1996, p. 544.

2. Peterson, D. "Hospital-Physician Relations: Beyond Courtship to the Ties That Bind." *HealthTexas,* Oct. 1991, p. 16.

3. Thompson, R. *Keys to Winning Physician Support.* Tampa, Fla.: American College of Physician Executives, 1993. p. 31.

Chapter 5
CHARACTERISTICS OF A SOUGHT-AFTER PRACTICING PHYSICIAN

A cooperative personality is almost as important as the other requirements. The medical staff is becoming more and more a group of physicians practicing together and uniting their efforts for patients' well-being. The physician who is an extreme individualist [can] cause friction and effectually prevent that cooperative action which is so necessary to efficiency. Such men [sic] should be refused membership on the medical staff, regardless of their personal competence and ethical standing.[1]

Regardless of exact organizational structures, ownership, and financing, and no matter how sophisticated computer systems become, center stage in health care will always belong to knowledgeable, skilled, and committed clinicians.

Here, clinical teams help people maintain "wellness." There, a team of practitioners fights against time to delay a death (one never "saves a life"). And elsewhere, practicing physicians provide long term support to individuals made infirm by the normal aging process and, in today's world, sometimes unsupported by their families.

How tempting it is to end this chapter right here. How tempting to believe that all a physician must do to win a secure position on the medical staff of an IHCDS is to exhibit the well-known and time-honored nobility of the healing profession. How tempting, and how foolish. Today's sought-after physician must be much more than a skilled clinician.

Defining the "Quality Physician"

In the academic and philosophical world, debates about the meaning of "quality" will never end. How can one define, quantify, and judge such an ephemeral, ethereal, elusive concept?

But the real world demands a practical definition of "quality," as in "quality physician." And framing such a definition is not as difficult as the task first sounds. The key is to drop the controversial word, "quality," and to speak instead of characteristics exhibited by a "sought-after" physician. Sought-after means chosen both by those needing medical care and by organizational providers of such care.

Here, to help the practicing physician reader understand what it takes to be among the chosen in today's competitive environment, is a sample list of the characteristics of sought-after physicians. The physician reader and his or her colleagues and co-workers can use this list as a starting point for creating their own definition of a sought-after practicing physician. So can IHCDS management.

Characteristics exhibited by sought-after physicians include:

I. Dependable Clinical Knowledge and Skills

First and foremost, the sought-after practicing physician exhibits command of the subject matter of his or her chosen clinical field. In addition, if performing dangerous procedures on people is part of the physician's chosen field of practice, performance data (see Chapter 9) indicate good technical skills as well.

II. Availability to Those in Need of Medical Care Services

Excellent clinical skills are of no value to patients if they are not applied with care to each patient's unique needs. This includes providing the same care to patients whether it is two o'clock in the afternoon or two o'clock in the morning. And it includes either being available nights and weekends, or arranging for "coverage" by a practicing physician colleague with relevant clinical skills and experience.

One advantage of practicing in an integrated system is that arranging "coverage," once the responsibility of each individual practicing physician or physician group, is now handled by those scheduling the time of physicians practicing in the IHCDS. Of course, system executives and the board of directors must plan and pay a staff of practicing physicians that includes enough individuals of various specialties to allow for "time off."

Note another serendipitous outcome of this integrated coverage arrangement. It renders obsolete the need to spend weeks and months in "bylaws revision meetings," arguing over the "coverage" problem and trying to arrive at a resolution of the problem satisfactory to both practicing physicians and management.

III. Reasonable Accessibility to Other Members of the Patient Care Team

The sought-after physician does not routinely become frustrated when asked to provide more information to those interpreting x-rays, imaging studies, and laboratory results. He or she does not routinely express resentment at being "interrupted" when a nurse asks to express a concern or needs a question answered. And he or she is not routinely "too busy" to provide in-service and orientation sessions to nurses and clinical technicians when invited to do so.

The word, "routinely," is important. We all have "bad hair days," when so much is going wrong that our reserves are exhausted. At that point, asking us to deal with one more question or concern, large or small, brings us to the boiling point, or even causes us to explode. When that happens to a usually reasonable and cooperative physician, co-workers should seek to understand whatever pressures the practicing physician is feeling, rather than making an immediate moral judgment ("Why is he so uncaring and insensitive?") or immediately assuming that the practitioner has suddenly become "impaired."

IV. Appreciation that Written Records Are Necessary

Few physicians enjoy keeping written records. Maintaining a balanced checkbook (manually or on a computer) is no more fun than completing patients' medical records (manually or on a computer). However, the sought-after physician accepts the need for good written records, for his or her protection as well as for the good of the patient and the IHCDS.

Take a "pretend you are the patient" approach to medical records. That mind-set helps one remember the need to someday recall accurately what happened to this patient being cared for by this team of practitioners at this point in time.

The IHCDS should establish systems that make the record-keeping task as simple as possible. Practicing physicians and others are greatly aided, for example, by a unit patient record. "Unit record" means that a patient or family's record of care from all system components is recorded in a single place. Computer networks make this possible.

It is unfair to ask practicing physicians to provide continuity of care without immediate access to up-to-date information about this specific patient.

"Completing" the Medical Record: Expect New Approaches

Traditional attempts to motivate physicians to complete the medical records of hospitalized patients have been ludicrous. Medical staff bylaws traditionally contain punitive-sounding threats about what will happen to a practicing physician who does not complete relevant portions of the medical record.

Through the years, "medical records librarians," who became medical records professionals and are now "specialists in health information systems," found themselves forced to engage in demeaning behavior. Within the past year, the author has witnessed the spectacle of a medical records specialist on duty at the door of an auditorium as physicians filed into a general medical staff meeting. Standing beside a cart full of incomplete patient records, the task of the medical records specialist was to buttonhole physicians and humorously plead for record entries and signatures. One physician who asked why his signature was so important was told only, "The Joint Commission says we have to get you to sign."

These traditional approaches have treated physicians like spoiled children, rather than as highly educated adults who must accept the responsibility of completing the patient's medical record, for their own sake as well as everybody else's.

Other New Approaches

New approaches will not be limited to new kinds of efforts to get physicians to write or dictate record entries and affix required signatures. Here are five examples:

- Each patient's record traditionally contains an "order sheet." And, traditionally, only physicians (and authorized physician's assistants) could write "orders." This prerogative is closely guarded by physician interest groups. One major task in "completing" a patient's record is to get attending and consulting physicians to authorize, in writing, orders that were given orally during the patient's care.

   Watch for well-qualified practitioners other than physicians to be given, by boards of directors (including physicians, remember), the prerogative to write on the order sheet.

   Watch for insurance company rules, relevant institutional licensing statutes, and Joint Commission standards to support this change.

   Also, watch for "the order sheet" to be given a less pejorative name, such as "prescribed patient care services."

- Watch for physicians to lose the prerogative of being the only individuals allowed to complete the "face sheets" of medical records. In an integrated system, there is little need for a medical record to be held up for the attention and the signature of a busy practicing physician.

Even with advances such as computer networking capabilities and increased acceptance of physician signature stamps, it makes sense for a team including clinical department chairs and physician executives, working with knowledgeable and skilled medical information specialists, to complete "face sheet" information.

- Watch for a dawning realization that retrospective authorization of verbal orders is not patient-protective. It is only provider-protective. Watch for greater demands that authorization of verbal orders be concurrent (by the nurse actually administering a medication, before the medication is given).

- Practicing physicians will find it easier in the immediate future (which has already arrived at some medical centers) to add notes and signatures to a patient's medical record. That's because computers in the physician's outpatient practice location are networking with computerized records of all kinds in other components of the IHCDS. This is one more good use for e-mail messages.

- Finally, look for system management (physician executives, remember) to be less accepting of excuses for not completing patient records in a timely fashion. There will be few justifiable reasons for hundreds of patient records to be incomplete on any given day in the various patient care components of the IHCDS.

The System's insistence that practicing physicians complete patient's records will no longer be a matter of coaxing and cajoling, or of threatening sanctions described in medical staff bylaws. Completing patient records will be a condition of employment or contract. (This trend was actually begun, amazingly enough, by activist physicians and their attorneys, who succeeded in getting medical staff bylaws provisions, such as those requiring completion of patient records, recognized by law in some states as contract obligations).

V. Understanding Acceptance of Responsibility in a Team Context

In some patient care circumstances, such as in the operating room or in stabilizing a critically ill patient, practicing physicians will continue to make immediate decisions and "order" the activities of other members of the patient care team. But in a much larger number of day-to-day "routine" patient care encounters, the sought-after physician is one who works well as a team member with other practitioners, such as nurses, therapists, pharmacists, and technicians.

The sought-after practicing physician exercises patience in helping other team members understand the physician's role in this particular patient's care. At the same time, the practicing physician listens patiently as other team members explain their roles and how the physician(s) on this case can make everyone's tasks easier to accomplish.

VI. Efficient Practice Habits

Efficient practice should be defined, in a written system policy, as primary concern for achieving good results of care from the viewpoint of the users of medical care services, with simultaneous attention to avoiding unnecessary services that do not contribute to the patient's medical outcome.

This policy should express concern about unnecessary patient discomfort when unneeded medical care is ordered, in addition to viewing overutilization from the standpoint of reducing costs. The policy should also reflect the fact that "efficiency" in medical practice is an acceptable concept that differs markedly from the unacceptable concept of "economy" in medical practice. Here is an example of the difference:

Efficiency — A 43-year-old man with a bone tumor was returned to productive living as inexpensively as possible. However, this was not a small tumor in the long bone of an adolescent boy with no secondary medical problems. This was a tennis-ball-sized tumor invading nerve roots in a man with a prior history of diabetes mellitus, hypertension, and abnormal renal function studies.

The cost of treating this patient was $126,000. Because the good result of care could not have been achieved without all medical services that were provided to the patient, it is agreed that guidelines for efficient treatment were met.

Economy — We'll do the best we can for this poor 43-year-old man with a bone tumor. But, because we need to maximize investor profit, we can only afford to give him four days of radiation therapy. If he needs an operation, he can have one, but only a 38-minute operation. At the end of 38 minutes, a member of the FCO (Financial Concerns Office) staff will step into the O.R. and cut out the lights.

Note: If rationing of health care services becomes the law of the land, economy in health care will be the prevailing notion and careful definitions of efficiency will be unnecessary.

VII. Attention to, without Feeling Totally Constrained by, Practice Guidelines

For a detailed discussion of this point, see Chapter 7.

General Characteristics

In addition to these seven specific characteristics related to clinical practice, the sought-after physician will display desirable personal traits and skills, including integrity, vision, and the ability to communicate well orally and in writing.

A Prediction about Selection of Practicing Physicians by an IHCDS

The profit-taking health care model has spawned an entire "physician recruiting" industry. However, a general trend in the United States today is to recognize overreliance on third parties in such matters as employment, contracts, and negotiations between organizations and individuals. Watch for less use of physician recruiting firms in the future.

This does not mean that we will ever return to the day when each practicing physician or physician group assumed the prerogative and the responsibility of bringing new physicians into the community. It means that system management will use the system's practicing physicians rather than physician recruiters to identify sought-after newly trained physicians, or physicians practicing elsewhere, to fill vacant slots on the medical staff.

Reference

1. Ponton, T. *The Medical Staff in the Hospital*, First Edition. Chicago, Ill. Physicians' Record Company, 1939, p. 49.

Chapter 6
ORDER-GIVER VS. TEAM PLAYER

So what can we expect in the next phase of U.S. health care's overhaul?

[One thing is] Responsibility downloaded—
doctors to nurses, nurses to technicians,
technicians to paraprofessionals, etc.[1]

There was a time when it was appropriate for the physician to be the unquestioned captain of the ship in all matters related to caring for patients. But that was a time when patient care system components included only the doctor, the patient, the nurse, clinical support personnel (laboratory, radiology, anesthesiology), administrative support, and an owner-appointed board of trustees.

Today, some additional people must be added to that list. Most notable are a variety of specialist and subspecialist clinical professionals. Practicing physicians in most specialties now depend on highly trained imaging technicians; technicians skilled in invasive procedures, such as in the cardiac catheterization unit ("heart cath lab"); and physicians' assistants.

Staffs of therapists and trainers help people maintain "wellness." Clinical specialists in addition to physicians tend to the mental and emotional health of people with chronic medical conditions, family members of the ill and elderly, and people with social diseases such as AIDS and chemical dependency.

In addition, clinical support services, such as "medical record-keeping," have become much more sophisticated. It's true we've gone overboard, building large staffs to maintain all kinds of relatively useless data. But today, a sought-after physician (see Chapter 5) would never dream of trying to practice without sophisticated, computerized documentation aids.

The fact is, then, that today's physician works with and depends on professionals and technicians who know more about some specialized aspects of providing medical care services than the physician does.

Example

The author can't help remembering that he was given much of the credit for establishing, some years ago, one of the first newborn intensive care units in a nonuniversity setting. In reality, the credit belongs to Billie Abron, RN (God's gift to sick newborns); respiratory therapist George Cussell; and a staff of nurses, aides, and technicians who made newborn intensive care a profession as opposed to just a job.

In addition, a great deal of credit goes to a medical center executive staff that appreciated the community's need for this medical care service, and its positive public relations value, in spite of the fact that the NICU consumed money and people resources rather than contributing directly to the medical center's profit margin.

No, the technology available today cannot be applied to patients by a single individual physician, no matter how skilled that physician is. "Managed care" of individual patients by teams traveling critical pathways would be a reality today, even if integration had not been complicated by various organizational acronyms and initialisms in the private sector and by political maneuvering in the public sector.

It's time to acknowledge...

Today, it is only appropriate for the physician to be the unquestioned captain of the ship in a crisis situation, such as a life-threatening medical emergency. In most other patient care situations, the practicing physician is now more like the CEO of a patient's care, coordinating and directing the proper choice and use of a vast array of available medical diagnostic and treatment modalities.

The "attending physician" is still captain of the ship in the sense that, like any CEO, he or she must accept the responsibility for all decisions made and implemented in the course of caring for a patient. But, like any good CEO, the responsible practicing physician must weigh input from and acknowledge critical contributions by a number of other individuals.

Thus, in the IHCDS, even as it is appropriate for management to speak of practicing physicians as participating partners, it is at the same time appropriate to speak of the practicing physician's partners in clinical care.

The Practicing Physician's Partners in Clinical Care

The practicing physician's partners in care include executive/management staff; clinical care personnel, such as nurses, aides, technicians, and therapists; patients and family members; and physician colleagues.

Executive/Management Staff

Entire books have been written about the "physician-CEO-board interface." Indeed, the author has written some of them.[2,3,4] Fortunately, such books are becoming obsolete as physician executives effectively bridge the gap between health care professionals with clinical backgrounds and those with business management backgrounds. (For a discussion of participation by practicing physicians in organizational decision-making, see Chapter 10.)

In addition, both management and practicing physicians benefit from doctors' efforts to complete each patient's medical record (manual or electronic) in a timely and accurate fashion, accept the responsibility of analyzing information to assist the performance improvement office, and recognize skilled and qualified nurse managers as full partners in patient care.

Other Members of the Clinical Care Team

Technical aspects of care are often left to specialist and subspecialist clinicians other than physicians in highly specialized areas such as cardiac surgery, medical intensive care units, renal dialysis, newborn ICUs, and diagnostic imaging centers.

In addition, there is a less specialized aspect of clinical teamwork, critically important to patients and family members, that received hardly any attention until the age of continuous quality improvement. That is, careful attention to the countless "handoffs" between various individuals caring for a single patient.

The IHCDS usually has dependable players at each skill position (although too few in some of today's health care conglomerates, downsized to maximize profit for investors). But patients may be ill-served (and malpractice suits may be filed) when people with impeccable technical skills and qualifications do not communicate well with one another and thus fumble the ball.

Example 1: The patient has just been told by his orthopedic surgeon that immediate surgery is necessary to correct the cruciate ligament tear in the knee suffered in the automobile accident. The doctors, nurses, and family members have now left the patient's room. Enter a bright and cheery aide carrying a lunch tray. "I'll bet you're hungry, aren't you? You're going to like this." "Thanks," says the patient, preoccupied with matters of importance beyond having lunch, "but I'm NPO."

"You are?" beams the aide. "That's so nice. You have a nice lunch now." (Exit cheery aide.)

Example 2: Following the surgery, the patient's orthopedist insisted that painful exercises be done four times a day, without fail. "Physical therapy will take you down to their place three times a day," explained the orthopedist. (I call physical therapists the physical terrorists. Deep down, though, I truly love 'em.) "Then, after your supper, ask the floor nurse for your leg weights, and just do the exercises yourself. Good healing and timely discharge from the hospital depend on this."

OK, the patient can do that. So, after supper, he asks the nurse for leg weights. The reply is...any guesses? "What leg weights?"

This response is not a confidence builder and actually creates suspicion and a very guarded patient attitude if anything goes wrong, whether it's the hospital's or doctor's fault or not.

Example 3: Following back surgery to remove a giant cell tumor, the patient presents himself as an outpatient to the radiology and imaging department for follow-up x-rays of the lumbo-sacral area. Noting a mistake by the radiology department clerk, the patient advises the x-ray technician, "There's a mistake on my requisition. I'm here for views of my lumbar spine, not my cervical spine.

"That's OK," calls the busy technician over her shoulder as she disappears down the hall to do something important. "Don't worry about it. They're both the same price."

Have a nice day.

If I had the authority to replace a lot of useless statistics with one truly useful data item, my choice would be a subset of incident reports and risk management data. This data item would sound a little like a football stat. It would be called "number of fumbles per patient."

Effective integration of medical care services among physicians and other clinical practitioners, and among components of the IHCDS, can reduce that statistic to nearly zero, to the benefit of the system and all its clinical practitioners, not to mention the benefit to the users of medical care services.

Patients and Family Members

Today's integrated systems serve a knowledgeable, consumer-oriented public. Every practicing physician must become skilled at explaining and negotiating specific care plans, or learn to delegate this task to trusted co-workers. Sometimes partnering with the patient is simply a matter of negotiating medication for a chronic problem.

Example: When my blood pressure reached the point I needed it, Al Eaddy (my excellent internist) put me on a beta-blocker plus a diuretic, every day. A few months later, Al became concerned about a high-normal uric acid and suggested stopping the diuretic. (Note the word, "suggested." One mark of an excellent internist is that Al knows when to suggest and when to give his patient no choice. He's good at both).

Two weeks later, I called him. "Look, Al," says I, "I know how I was feeling when you first put me on high blood pressure meds, and I'm feeling that way again. I want that diuretic back. I don't see why I should give up feeling good just because you're concerned about some lab result."

I got my diuretic back. But only every other day. And only after promising to take time to get a stress test.

This was good negotiating by Al. (And by me, too. This way, I can still eat gobs of potato chips. At least on diuretic days.)

Any good practicing physician learns to negotiate such compromises, to increase the chances of patient compliance with prescribed regimens. This is a critical part of clinical practice not yet fully understood and acknowledged by advocates of too-compulsive adherence to practice guidelines.

But in other scenarios, the physician/patient/family negotiation process is much more serious. And emotionally draining. For example, today's practicing physician (and his or her family) must deal with the strain of helping patients (and their families) choose among complex treatment (or nontreatment) options made available by today's amazing technology. When the technology was not available, the choices did not exist. But today, the definition of "irreversible medical condition" is not always absolute.

"Irreversible" once really meant nothing could be done. Now, patients and family members and their attending and consulting physicians are faced with the fact that a condition may be "irreversible, except..." or "irreversible, unless...."

I write this chapter only a few days after involvement, as a friend with an MD degree, in helping a family/physician team arrive at a difficult decision. Cliff's bad, 80-year-old knees were replaced in surgery that was without complications in the first 72 hours postop. But then he developed adult respiratory insufficiency syndrome for reasons that are not entirely clear, even to his excellent team of physician and nurse specialists. He was placed on a respirator.

Over the next ten days, during which he received excellent supportive care, Cliff's lungs (described as "whited out" on x-ray) and blood gasses did not improve. The clinical team (not just the nurses but the physician as well) were extremely good to take time to advise Cliff's wife of his condition and possible complications. And they were sensitive enough to discover that their patient's wife was agonizing over the fact that the patient had insisted several times on strict adherence to provisions of his living will. "I'm not sure he'd be wanting us to put him through this," she said, although the patient was of course kept sedated and unconscious so as not to fight the respirator.

When Cliff's kidneys failed, with continued worsening of the lung picture, the physicians and nurses respected the family's choice to discontinue the respirator rather than to pursue further extraordinary efforts to prolong life.

The challenge for today's and tomorrow's practicing physician is to welcome the role of patients and family members in deciding their own fate. Meeting this challenge requires that the practicing physician develop three attitudes. The first is the willingness to share useful information with patients and families, so that their decision can be reasoned and valid. The second is the ability to support a family in a decision with which the physician may not fully agree. The third attitude is feeling professional satisfaction, not from assuming that one is all-knowledgable and all-powerful, but from understanding that patients and family members need continued participation and support from their physicians when death is imminent and inevitable.

Furthermore, practicing physicians must participate in discussions under way to more carefully consider the impact on people's lives of the ability to provide so much medical technology. We (the medical care system) played God at the point of having the technology to fix those darned knees. We played God when we put Cliff on a respirator. And we play God to the point of honoring Living Wills. How much longer can we avoid the responsibility of going one step further and allowing people and family members to decide whether some fates are not indeed worse than death? When one's beliefs make earth-life-end a religious issue, those religious beliefs must be respected. But many religious individuals embrace a faith that allows the medical care system to be of assistance when pain and suffering from an irreversible medical condition make death an option preferable to continued earthly existence.

Watch for the term "assisted suicide" to be dropped, in favor of a less pejorative term. Watch for professional religionists and ethicists to be sought after in professional and policy-making forums where divergent discussion is one day replaced by convergence on a national policy respecting death as everyone's ultimate destination.

One cannot imagine these critical discussions occurring without the full participation, if not leadership, of actively practicing physicians.

Note that the challenge for the practicing physician in this emotionally intense area has little to do with faddish organizational acronyms and issues of ownership and health care financing mechanisms. With the support of IHCDS management, the practicing physician can now use time once spent on administrative red tape to focus on critical, clinical, real-world issues.

Colleagues (Clinical Consultants)

Clinical consultants are very important partners in clinical care. It's taken for granted that every practicing physician knows how to seek and use clinical consultation. In reality, working with a clinical consultant is an underdeveloped art.

When

It's usually accepted by practicing physicians that clinical consultation is indicated when:

- The diagnosis is obscure after the results of initial diagnostic studies are known.

- Contemplated procedures or treatments place the patient at high risk.

- The patient's response to treatment seems delayed beyond the time when most patients can be expected to show improvement.

- The patient develops unexpected complications.

- The patient is in a special care unit, being cared for by a physician whose level of experience and training is less than that of readily available specialists and subspecialists in specific clinical areas related to intensive care of a patient's condition.

Consultation is requested by the patient and/or the patient's responsible family members.

Who

Choice of consultants by patients and family members, and by the attending physician, may or may not be more limited in the integrated system than in the old "freestanding private practice" system, depending on the local setting.

In the old system, patient choice was limited by referring relationships between individual practitioners. And the primary physician's choice of clinical consultant was limited by the choice of hospital attachment exercised by specialists.

In an integrated system, the choice of clinical consultants is dictated by system management, through the contract or hiring mechanism by which the medical staff is selected. One of the most measurable "quality" features of an IHCDS is the ready availability of appropriate, timely clinical consultation by highly qualified practitioners.

So this is an area where management knows it cannot afford to be Scrooge-like.

By the way, the belief that total "free choice" is a key to good medical care is a myth promulgated by those who benefit from the system of free choice of physician.

A responsible attending physician should, and usually does, guide the patient and family members to accept a clinical consultant whose track record is known to and acceptable to the "referring physician." Careful selection of the integrated system's physician panel actually may increase a particular patient's chances of being matched with a highly qualified specialist consultant.

How

When a clinical consultant is asked to see a patient, it is imperative that division of responsibility between the attending physician and consulting physician(s) be clarified. Such clarification is necessary to protect the patient, to avoid frustration and errors by nurses and others caring for the patient, to let nurses and others caring for the patient know whom to call if the patient presents a medical or surgical emergency, and to protect both the attending and consulting physician(s) from the legal consequences of embarrassing oversights or lack of communication about who is primarily responsible for the patient at each point in the patient's care.

Figure 6-1, page 46, (or a computerized version) can be completed and placed in the patient's medical record when clinical consultation is ordered.

Clinical Support Services

The attending physician must provide needed information to clinical care partners, such as pathologists, the clinical laboratory, radiology and imaging, and anesthesiology. A lengthy treatise here is unlikely to accomplish what is better accomplished by on-site, one-on-one motivation and training of attending physicians by statesman-like clinical support physicians.

References

1. Sheehy, B., and others. "Don't Blink or You'll Miss It: The Reformation of U.S. Healthcare Is Under Way." *The Medical Leadership Forum.* La Jolla, Calif., Fall 1995, page 16.

2. Thompson, R. *Helping Trustees Understand Physicians.* Chicago, Ill.: American Hospital Association, 1979.

3. Thompson, R. *Physicians and Hospitals: Easing Adversary Relationships.* Chicago, Ill.: Pluribus Press, 1984.

4. Thompson, R. *Keys to Winning Physician Support.* Tampa, Fla.: American College of Physician Executives, 1991.

Figure 6-1.

REQUEST FOR CLINICAL CONSULTATION

To be completed and placed in the patient's medical record when clinical consultation is ordered:

Date of Request _____

Date of Initial Patient Visit by Clinical Consultant _____

Attending (Requesting) Physician_____

Clinical Consultant_____

The following information is to be completed by the Requesting Physician.

Reason(s) for requesting clinical consultation:

[ ] Diagnosis obscure.

[ ] Need assessment of patient's risk with respect to contemplated diagnostic and therapeutic procedures.

[ ] Patient not responding to treatment as expected.

[ ] Patient has developed (an) unexpected complication(s).

[ ] The patient is in a special care unit, being cared for by a physician with less than Level 3 clinical privileges in the relevant clinical area(s).

[ ] Patient or family requests clinical consultation.

[ ] Need a second opinion.

[ ] Other_____

Please

[ ] Evaluate the patient and discuss findings and suggestions with me, OR;

[ ] Evaluate the patient, discuss findings and suggestions with me, and follow with me, OR;

[ ] Assume care of the patient.

_____
Requesting Physician (Signature)

┌Chapter 7
THE PROPER USE OF PRACTICE GUIDELINES

Physicians have long adhered to critical pathways of sorts.... Why do we have only one pediatric immunization schedule for every person on the planet? Because it works....

What has worked so effectively in the realm of public health is also working today in private practice.[1]

See the Glossary for a distinction between practice guidelines and critical pathways. This chapter focuses on the use of practice guidelines.

A complete treatise on practice guidelines is beyond the intended scope of this book. The purpose of this chapter is simply to suggest that there are good ways and bad ways for practicing physicians to use practice guidelines in integrated systems, and to suggest which is which.

The physician reader will already be well aware of the points made in this chapter. The author suggests that physicians share this chapter with management-trained individuals who need a better understanding of the realities of clinical decision-making in the context of caring for an individual patient.

The care of individual patients can be standardized more than some physicians yet understand and accept. But variation cannot be reduced to the extent wished for by some proponents of practice guidelines. Participation in cooperative efforts to blend these two viewpoints is one of the most important challenges facing physicians practicing in systems.

Practice guidelines are bad when they are used only to focus on the organization's interest in this quarter's (financial) bottom line. Practice guidelines are also bad when there is an attempt to depend on these care templates as absolute standards from which a practitioner should not deviate.

These two abuses of practice guidelines (total obsession with cost and taking an approach that is too absolute) can be avoided with a little thought and practice. So they are not arguments against using practice guidelines. Practice guidelines are an excellent concept when used with attention to delivering dependable medical care to each patient, being concerned with cost-effectiveness within that context, and when reasonable flexibility is allowed.

Square Pegs and Round Holes

Flexibility in applying practice guidelines is necessary because people who can be lumped together in broad categories ("heart attack," "diabetes," "high blood pressure," "kidney infection," "chest pain," "low back pain," "dysfunctional uterine bleeding," "ulcer," etc.) are really unique individuals who do not have the same body reactions to either a given disease process or its accepted treatment.

Individual differences to be considered in this context include physical differences, emotional differences, differences in the degree of patient compliance, and differences in how soon medical attention is sought.

Physical Differences

Have you ever noticed a stranger who is a dead ringer for a friend? Do you remember your reaction? It was surprise. ("He looks just like Bill!") Look around the room during a dead spot in your next meeting. Do you see two persons with absolutely identical facial characteristics? Not unless there are identical twins in the room.

The body's reactions to disease and treatment are as unique as one's facial characteristics. In pediatric practice, the same medication prescribed for three different children might produce the desired result in one, an unexpected and undesirable reaction in another, and a complaint from the parent of the third child that money was wasted on a prescription that had no effect on the child at all.

Emotional Differences

Unfortunately for the doctor, people differ in their ability to differentiate pain and fatigue that are a normal part of everyone's life from nature's warnings about serious medical problems. A hypochondriac views every doctor as being callous and uncaring. On the other hand, a stoic person can make a doctor look bad when a diagnosis is made that was missed earlier because the stoic person's perception of severe pain warning of a serious condition was "a little discomfort."

Differences in Patient Compliance

A few minutes and a brief explanation, using standard written instructions, may be enough for one patient to be trained and motivated to comply with prescribed diet, activity, and medication regimens. Another person may do better if the information can be viewed on videotape. But for the next patient, achieving compliance may require lengthy explanations with, "Repeat that back to me again," and repetitive one-on-one educational sessions, all combined with efforts to motivate the patient to comply. Language barriers and educational differences are only the most visible of many factors accounting for these individual differences. So, even in a matter as seemingly simple as "patient instruction," absolute guidelines will not suffice.

Differences in How Soon Help Is Sought

The doctor may first see a patient early in the course of a medical problem, or too late to avoid complications that could have been avoided if the patient sought medical attention earlier. The need to tailor specific patient care plans to a time-point in the natural history of an illness is only superficially acknowledged in practice guidelines at this early stage of their development.

Some Principles for Using Practice Guidelines

Practicing physicians; clinical leaders, such as chairs of clinical departments or medical service areas; performance improvement office personnel; and system executive staff and board should memorialize key principles in a "Practice Guidelines Policy."

The purpose of practice guidelines is to respond to the following question: "Do diagnostic and treatment modalities selected for this patient match this individual's specific patient care needs, yet reduce variation to the extent desirable and possible?"

This statement of purpose suggests the following definition and system policy:

- "Practice guidelines are systematically developed statements to assist practitioner and patient decisions about appropriate health care for specific clinical circumstances."

- "Attention to practice guidelines is encouraged, with the under standing that they are not absolute. That is, in the course of individual-clinical-decision making, deviations from practice guidelines should be expected. In that event, it is in the practitioner's best interest to carefully note, in the patient's record, the clinical reason(s) that generally stated practice guidelines do not effectively meet the patient's specific needs."

- "As part of physician performance improvement activities [see Chapter 9], data should be developed that are useful in identifying:

  ▸ Appropriate use of practice guidelines.

  ▸ The need to further examine a physician's significant and/or frequent departure from well-accepted practice guidelines."

Three keys to successful use of practice guidelines are:

- Pay as much attention to using practice guidelines in the interest of good patient results as to furthering the organization's interest in staying within budget and/or maximizing investor profit;

- Distinguish between the use of guidelines, criteria, standards, and performance indicators.

  The following definitions are useful when properly understood and reflected in implementation.[2]

  Practice guidelines are systematically developed statements to assist practitioner and patient decisions about appropriate health care for specific clinical circumstances.

  Performance measures (provisional definition) are methods or instruments to estimate or monitor the extent to which the actions of a health care practitioner or provider conform to practice guidelines, medical review criteria, or standards of quality.

  Medical review criteria are systematically developed statements that can be used to assess the appropriateness of specific health care decisions, services, and outcomes.

  Standards of quality are authoritative statements of minimum levels of acceptable performance of results, of excellent levels of performance or results, or of the range of acceptable performance or results.

One underlying premise highlighted by these definitions is that the four terms are not synonymous. Assisting physicians, nurses, other practitioners, and patients in making decisions (through practice guidelines) is not the same as evaluating practice (using medical review criteria, standards of quality, and performance measures). Therefore, although the definitions may further evolve, it is important to underscore (retain the principle) that the phrases and concepts are not equivalent and should not be used interchangeably.

- Avoid too absolute an approach. In previous years, unnecessary conflict has been created by treating statements intended as professional and organizational guidelines as though they were absolute legal standards.

References

1. Musfeldt, C. "Outpatient Critical Pathways: Five Advantages for Physicians Who Act Now." *Physician Executive* 22(4):10-1, April 1996.

2. Field, M., and Lohr, K., Editors. *Clinical Practice Guidelines, Directions for a New Program.* Washington, D.C.: National Academy Press, 1990, pp. 8-9.

Chapter 8

CREDENTIALING IN THE INTEGRATED HEALTH CARE DELIVERY SYSTEM

The word "staff" is defined for the purposes of this chapter as the group of doctors who practice in the hospital, inclusive of the "regular staff," "the visiting staff," the "associate staff," and other designated physician categories.

"Membership upon the staff [is] restricted to physicians and surgeons who are (a) full graduates of medicine in good standing and legally licensed to practice in their respective states and provinces, (b) competent in their respective fields, and (c) worthy in character and in matters of professional ethics; in this/latter connection, the practice of the division of fees, under any guise whatever, [is] prohibited.[1]

Credential—That which certifies one's authority or claim to confidence. (Related to "credibility," which is "the capacity of being believed.")[2]

Physician credentialing is concerned with a practicing physician's qualifications. For a discussion of methods and activities related to confirming current dependable performance, see Chapter 9.

Once upon a time, a practicing physician chose a community in which to work, established an office, and immediately applied to each hospital in town for the privilege of using that hospital's services for his or her sickest patients.

Before granting that privilege, the hospital (physician leaders, administration, and board of trustees) checked out the physician's basic credentials. These included medical school diploma; specialty residency if any; state licensure; registration to dispense narcotics; and, in more recent years, malpractice experience.

The exact process for each physician applicant differed according to the amount of experience the applicant had accumulated. If the physician was just out of training, the credentialing inquiry was of necessity limited to validating formal training. If the physician had previously practiced in another location, "reference letters" were a major part of the credentialing process.

In theory, the board of trustees appointed the medical staff. In reality, boards usually rubber-stamped the decisions of local practicing physicians doubling as hospital "organized medical staff" leaders.

Sometimes physicians attempted to commandeer the credentialing process for economic reasons, such as to exclude potential competitors. Contaminating the patient-protective credentialing process with such economic considerations was frowned upon.

Also, note the admonition against fee splitting in the initial description of a hospital credentialing system (see above). The intent was not only to avoid unnecessary costs for the patient (third-party payment is a relatively recent development), but also to ensure that physician decisions and actions were based on need, not on maximizing revenue for physicians. (Concern about fee-splitting is reflected in modern times by the concern that decisions and actions of physicians and hospitals in certain kinds of economic relationships might be based on maximizing profit, rather than on patient need.)

The "pure" patient-protective system just described was designed for a time when the hospital was a professional community institution established by a combination of philanthropists and civic leader physicians. In that system, the hospital's purpose was simple: To provide the town's practicing physicians with suitable facilities and support to care for seriously ill patients. In fact, axioms of the time included, "The hospital is the doctor's workshop" and "Never forget that your real customer is the doctor."

In the 1980s and early 1990s, the credentialing system was different. Contamination of credentialing decisions by economic considerations ("economic credentialing") was openly encouraged. That's because the avowed purpose of emerging conglomerates was clearly different than the purpose of yesterday's community hospital. That avowed goal was to "maximize investor profit." Satisfaction of public need and providing the physician with needed space, equipment, and clinical support staff to provide safe and effective patient care were pursued only as far as was deemed necessary within that context.

But in today's integrated systems, the pendulum is swinging toward balanced attention to both profit and provision of dependable patient care services. So the credentialing system currently evolving simultaneously serves the needs of the public, practicing physicians, and the integrated system itself.

Three-Dimensional Credentialing

In the IHCDS, the design and implementation of procedures for confirming a practicing physician's entry-level qualifications ("credentialing") must simultaneously achieve three distinct objectives:

- Protect patients by focusing attention on physician qualifications from the viewpoint of individuals needing medical care (patients and family members).

- Protect practicing physicians by creating a positive public image, building a practice (being a sought-after provider by both IHCDSs and their individual beneficiaries), and avoiding legal misadventures.

- Protect the integrated system by creating a positive public image; building a practice (being the provider organization chosen by those with money seeking to contract for the delivery of medical care services); avoiding legal misadventures; and, within the context of those goals, choosing physicians who practice efficiently.

Physician credentialing remains particularly important in the acute care component of the integrated system. While system leaders may wish to focus on "wellness" and cost concerns, patients and the community of potential patients focus on whether or not they receive dependable medical care on the scariest days of their "covered lives."

Credentialing Methods and Tools

Specific methods for credentialing physicians in managed care settings are still evolving.

In one IHCDS, the practicing physician may encounter credentialing methods that are little more than expansions of the overly complex, legalistic credentialing systems of acute care hospitals in the 1970s and 1980s (ancient history in the context of today's rapidly evolving integrated clinical practice settings).

But in another IHCDS, the practicing physician may be pleased to find innovative approaches to credentialing using "new paradigm" (fundamentally changed) credentialing tools and methods. The change is not so much in the structure of credentialing tools (application forms, validation requests, etc.) as in the handling of accumulated information about an applicant to achieve the three goals listed above.[3,4]

For example, the decision about whether the applicant may participate (be a "medical staff member," be on a "physician panel," etc.) may be handled by one group, while the question of whether or not the physician's professional qualifications are adequate may be handled by another. The criteria used by the first group may be system-component specific, but the criteria used to determine professional qualifications must be the same for all system components to avoid a "double standard" in patient care.

Furthermore, IHCDS leaders implementing credentialing methods will not be primarily concerned with requirements of external licensing and accrediting bodies. Complying with regulations and standards will be a secondary concern, which can usually be met by pro forma activities ("going through the motions"). But the primary concern of the successful IHCDS is genuine, substantive decision making based on careful analysis of submitted information, to achieve the three goals of the credentialing process stated above.

Structure and Information Flow in IHCDS Physician Credentialing

Figure 8-1 shows a schematic summary of one possible way to avoid duplication of effort and to clarify relative authority and responsibility while accomplishing effective IHCDS Credentialing. It is not intended that the reader should photocopy and adopt this plan. Rather, the author's hope is that this template diagram will help the reader discover the IHCDS credentialing plan that is most effective for his or her particular setting.

The plan depicted in figure 8-1 is based on the following assumptions:

1. The three purposes and goals of the credentialing process are those stated on page 55.

2. At the present time, decision makers in each system component wish to retain their authority, as opposed to relinquishing credentialing authority and responsibility to an overall system board.

3. Credentialing procedures and decisions must be fair to practitioners.

4. Credentialing must be accomplished as efficiently as possible, within the reality of several clinical practice locations and several layers of management within the system.

5. #2 can be accomplished without duplicating committees and without duplicating steps, such as collecting and validating information provided in support of an application.

Figure 8-1

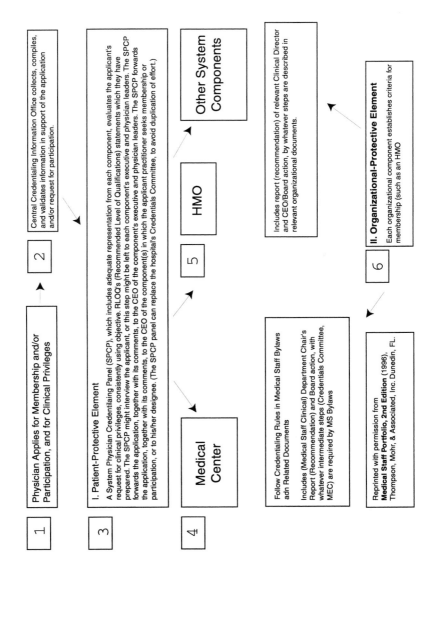

1 Physician Applies for Membership and/or Participation, and for Clinical Privileges

2 Central Credentialing Information Office collects, compiles, and validates information in support of the application and/or request for participation.

3 **I. Patient-Protective Element**

A System Physician Credentialing Panel (SPCP), which includes adequate representation from each component, evaluates the applicant's request for clinical privileges, consistently using objective, RLOQ's (Recommended Level of Qualifications) statements which they have prepared. The SPCP might interview the applicant, or this step might be left to each component's executive and physician leaders. The SPCP forwards the application, together with its comments, to the CEO of the component's executive and physician leaders. The SPCP forwards the application, together with its comments, to the CEO of the component(s) in which the applicant practitioner seeks membership or participation, or to his/her designee. (The SPCP panel can replace the hospital's Credentials Committee, to avoid duplication of effort.)

4 Medical Center

Follow Credentialing Rules in Medical Staff Bylaws adn Related Documents

Includes (Medical Staff Clinical) Department Chair's Report (Recommendation) and Board action, with whatever intermediate steps (Credentials Committee, MEC) are required by MS Bylaws

5 HMO

6 **II. Organizational-Protective Element**

Each organizational component establishes criteria for membership (such as an HMO

Includes report (recommendation) of relevant Clinical Director and CEO/Board action, by whatever steps are described in relevant organizational documents.

Other System Components

Reprinted with permission from **Medical Staff Portfolio, 2nd Edition** (1996), Thompson, Mohr, & Associated, Inc. Dunedin, FL.

CREDENTIALING IN THE INTEGRATED HEALTH CARE DELIVERY SYSTEM

6. The organization-protective element of physician credentialing can be component-specific as long as patient/public interests are as well-served as organizational interests. For example, if there is more than one hospital in the integrated system, clinical privileges might still follow the tradition of being "hospital-specific," based on differences in support staff and clinical equipment. These differences might relate to avoiding duplication for cost-saving purposes or to different missions of the hospitals that are part of the system, such as providing secondary rather than tertiary medical care services. Such efficiencies should be encouraged, rather than hindered, by public policy. And money saved should support maintenance of dependable medical services rather than being drained out of the system as investor profit.

7. In contrast, the patient-protective element of credentialing, which consists of awarding to each practicing physician specific clinical privileges matched to the level of the individual's training and qualifications, cannot be system-component specific. Rather, the IHCDS must ensure, insofar as is humanly possible, that patients with the same or similar medical needs receive the same dependable care in all components of the system presuming to offer the services of system physicians.

Implementation Aids

The following notes are intended to help relevant individuals understand and implement a plan such as that depicted in Figure 8-1. Each note pertains to a numbered element in Figure 8-1.

1. A central credentialing office should provide the applicant with all relevant forms pertaining to desired affiliations with system components, desired clinical practice locations within the system, and confirmation of the applicant's clinical training and experience in his or her declared specialty.

   The form designed or adopted to collect basic information about the applicant (such as training, licensure, etc.) may be the same for all components or may be modified by each component to suit that component's particular needs for specific relevant information. However, the same ISCP (individual-specific clinical privileges) application form should be given to all applicants practicing the same specialty or subspecialty in various organizational components and practice locations within the system.

2. Individuals staffing the central credentialing office are duly qualified individuals with relevant expertise in physician credentialing procedures. They may have served a similar function in a hospital/medical center. However, care should be taken to retrain these individuals so that IHCDS physician credentialing is not just an extension of the overly complex and legalistic activity in U.S. acute care hospitals in the 1970s and 1980s.

3. The heart of the patient-protective element of this managed care physician credentialing plan is the system physician credentialing panel (SPCP), appointed according to relevant descriptions and provisions in the system's governance documents. Physicians appointed to this panel should have a reputation for objectivity and fairness, good clinical skills, good communication skills, and experience in physician credentialing, such as in a hospital/medical center.

   The director (coordinator) of the central credentialing office serves as staff to the SPCP. This person handles the logistics of distributing each completed application, along with the SPCP's comments, to the CEOs of relevant components of the system or to their designees.

4. At this writing, consideration of and decisions on credentials applications in acute care hospitals/medical centers follow the traditional medical staff/board "two-bylaws system." This system is traditionally authorized in governing body bylaws and is described in detail in medical staff bylaws and related documents.

5. Decisions about participation in the clinical activities of other components of the system may relate to specific criteria for participation in some system component, such as an HMO, a multispecialty physician group, or an insurance company physician panel.

6. The specific criteria for membership or participation developed and used by each system component should include attention to cost concerns, public image, avoiding unnecessary duplication within the system, and legal liability. Even in this component of credentialing, success of the organization depends on making patient care considerations (such as the ability to provide dependable health care services to the entire community of potential patients who are members or beneficiaries of this system) the paramount concern.

References

1. *The Minimum Standard for Hospitals.* Chicago, Ill.: American College of Surgeons, 1919.

2. *Funk and Wagnall's New Comprehensive International Dictionary of the English Language.* Newark, N.J.: Publisher's International Press. Newark, 1980, p. 304.

3. Thompson, R. *The Medical Staff Leader's Practical Guidebook,* 3rd Edition. Marblehead, Mass.: Opus Publishers, 1996, Chapter 5, "Introduction to Credentialing," pp. 27-41.

4. Thompson, R. Medical Staff Portfolio, *Three-Part Credentialing Manual and Related Policies for Use,* 2nd Edition. Dunedin, Fla.: Thompson, Mohr, and Associates, Inc., 1996.

Chapter 9
CONFIRMING DEPENDABLE PERFORMANCE (QUALITY) OF ALL COMPONENTS OF THE IHCDS: THE PRACTICING PHYSICIAN'S ROLE

Forcing down costs is clearly today's top priority, but, over time (as costs come under control), quality will take precedence. When this shift occurs (and it will happen suddenly), those caught on the wrong side of the quality curve will suffer badly. This is not a hope or a threat, but a well-formed prediction.[1]

The fear engendered by the inspectors in a regulation-driven quality paradigm simply doesn't exist in quality environments responding primarily to economic pressures.[2]

The challenge of marketing in the 1990s, in all U.S. businesses, is to compete on the basis of quality as well as cost. (See figure 9-1, Page 62) It is unfortunate, therefore, that the past experience of today's health care leaders leaves them ill-prepared to put together positive "quality data" and inexperienced at sharing information of any kind with purchasers, payers, and the public.

The author's purpose in this book does not include reciting the past history of "quality assessment" and "evaluating physician performance." (For the interested reader, such histories are available.[3,4]) Suffice it to say that these terms, until recently, were euphemisms for negative, punitive efforts characterized by inefficient committee work, reams of essay-type "documentation," and legal tangles. Concern for keeping all "quality" information secret was a big feature of that era.

So today we are witnessing a paradox. On one hand, success of an IHCDS now depends partly on developing and sharing positive quality data. On the other hand, management leaders and physicians who are the transition group between yesterday and tomorrow are conditioned to believe that all "quality" data are negative and should be kept "confidential."

Figure 9-1

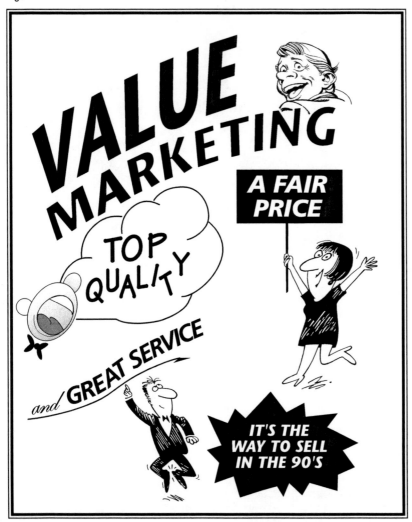

Example: The author recently conducted a physician leadership training seminar during which several key physician leaders became keenly interested in new, positive methods of drawing valid conclusions from performance data. Their interest was heightened by a physician leader of a new physician-hospital organization (PHO), who assured the physicians that, "This isn't just for the Joint Commission anymore; we'll be looking at such data to pick and keep doctors on our practice panel."

This physician group was discouraged, however, because it did not believe such data were readily available, and it believed that setting up a system to collect such data would be costly and impractical.

The author gave his usual explanation that it's a little late for objections based on the assumption that "this can't be done," because IHCDSs everywhere are collecting such data. Following the seminar, the CEO of the IHCDS asked to see the author in her office. There, telling me that this conversation must be kept strictly confidential, she showed me a collection of useful data of which she was justifiably quite proud. That means that the locally developed data system was impressive. But it also means that the data confirmed positive performance. The data include what the physicians need in order to proceed with meaningful "performance improvement" activities, which can be of great benefit to the IHCDS as well as to the physicians themselves and to the public served by the IHCDS. But this CEO was afraid to share any of the data, even positive data, with anyone, including her physician leaders.

The point is that concerns about "confidentiality" reached ridiculous extremes in the overly adversarial age of the 1980s and early 1990s.

The practicing physician/physician executive team is well-qualified to change the focus of evaluating physician performance from "policing" to developing and sharing positive data.[5] Here are nine keys to accomplishing this transformation.

Nine Keys

1. **State clear objectives**. Objectives of efforts to confirm consistently dependable performance include:

   ‣ Focus the attention of IHCDS executives, managers, all personnel, and practicing physicians, on promoting good patient care results.

   ‣ Focus public attention on the fact that dependable performance is actually the IHCDS's number one priority, not just a clever marketing gimmick.

   ‣ Enhance organizational productivity.

   Advertise the fact that internal evaluation of this information is now used as a basis for rewarding, retaining, and updating the continuing medical education of physicians on the IHCDS's practice panel, medical staff, and/or list of "preferred providers."

2. **Define "quality."** In a philosophy classroom, discussions of the elusive, ephemeral, ethereal nature of "quality" will continue forever. In the IHCDS, we can afford no such luxury. Success depends on defining "quality" as "confirmed dependable performance from the viewpoint

of users of medical care services, ranging from maintenance of good health through support of chronic medical conditions, and including dependable acute care on the scariest days of a person's covered life."

To avoid confusion, don't even use the term, "quality." Use the term "performance."

3. **Define the activities in which practicing physicians are expected to participate.** In the integrated system, all clinical components (acute critical and emergency care, long-term care, ambulatory care, mental health services, etc.) must develop and use information providing reassuring answers to at least four questions about dependable performance. Each of these performance questions can be matched to specific performance initiatives in the following manner:

▸ Performance Question #1. Do selected diagnostic and treatment modalities match individual patient needs, yet reduce variation to the extent desirable and possible?

▸ Performance Initiative #1. Reasonable use of practice guidelines.

▸ Performance Question #2. Is aggregate performance dependable?

▸ Performance Initiative #2. Drawing valid conclusions from reliable data concerning various statistical populations served by the IHCDS.

▸ Performance Question #3. Is individual performance dependable?

▸ Performance Initiative #3. This performance initiative has two parts, in the context of confirming dependable physician performance:

　1. (Confirming basic entry-level qualifications ("credentialing").

　2. (Confirming current dependable performance ("quality"), drawing valid conclusions from reliable data, and sharing this information in the form of physician performance reports.

▸ Performance Question #4. Are the systems, services, and communication aspects of patient care dependable?

▸ Performance Initiative #4. Physicians participate with nurses, other clinical personnel, and management to develop, implement, and maintain systems of dependable patient care. This is the activity once known as "total quality management."

　　This concept of four performance questions and matching performance initiatives can help relieve confusion about the relationship between such efforts as credentialing and use of physician performance information on one hand, and continuous quality improvement (CQI) attention to systems on the other.

4. **List important performance factors (characteristics of a sought-after physician).** For a sample list and relevant discussion, see Chapter 5.

5. **Understand the difference between use of practice guidelines, performance indicators, criteria, and standards** (See Chapter 7). Discuss the differences in using practice guidelines, performance indicators, criteria, and standards with colleagues and co-workers.

   Decide whether you agree with the statement that unnecessary problems have been caused in past years by the tendency to use statements intended as professional guidelines as though they were absolute legal standards.

   Now embody the results of your discussion in a formal, adopted policy on use of practice guidelines, performance indicators, criteria, and standards. You will find this clarification helpful in many ways. For example, practicing physicians must be participants in developing practice guidelines, but selecting good Indicators of performance may not require physician participation. That's because practice guidelines are intended to dictate behavior, whereas indicators of performance are simply answers to the question, "What is the simplest way to measure performance?"

   Example: Airline baggage handlers must participate in designing protocols for handling airline baggage (practice guidelines), but one doesn't have to be a baggage handler to understand that a good indicator of performance is the number and percentage of lost bags.

6. **Focus efforts on developing positive data.** In a written policy, state that the purpose of collecting, interpreting, and using performance data is to confirm dependable performance through the collection and sharing of relevant and useful information. The policy should include the statement that, if negative information emerges, positive efforts are taken to improve systems, educate and train physicians and personnel, and/or motivate improvement in an individual's performance, whatever the need.

   Subsequently, information that is now positive should be shared with payers and the public, along with the positive information that the IHCDS has established, and uses, mechanisms to improve both systems and individual performance when necessary. In designing your methods, be sure to focus on the positive approach. For example, if "patient complaints" is a useful indicator, so is "patient compliments."

A caveat. Don't throw out the baby with the bathwater. Maintain effective mechanisms for dealing with outlier behavior and performance by an irascible, recalcitrant individual unresponsive to positive efforts aimed at motivating the individual to voluntarily make necessary changes in behavior and/or performance.

7. **Draw valid conclusions.** "Interpreting data" means, to some, that statistics about what happens to groups of people or things are manipulated statistically. But one contribution of CQI advocates is to point out the critical importance of "cause and effect analysis" when drawing conclusions from data. This simply means asking and answering, "Why?"

When drawing a conclusion about whether or not a physician's performance is dependable, it is important not to skip the step of cause and effect analysis. One example is use of infection rates. "Hospital A's postop infection rate is 5 percent. Hospital B's postop infection rate is 10 percent. Therefore, one would rather be in Hospital A." With attention to some mitigating factors, this approach can work to evaluate and compare aggregate performance, without needing to define individual contributions to observed results.

It's tempting to simply apply the same method when the objective is to evaluate and compare individual performance. "Physician A's infection rate is 5 percent; physician B's infection rate is 10 percent. Therefore, physician A is a better, more careful clinician than physician B." That won't work, because the step of cause and effect analysis has been skipped. That is, physician performance is not the only factor contributing to the development of an infection or to a patient's dying. Why did the infection develop? When during the patient's course did the infection develop?

One orthopedic surgeon relates the experience of receiving a warning letter from "Infection Control" because of an infection in one of his patients. In actuality, the orthopedist was the last physician on the case and had to amputate the unfortunate patient's leg because of uncontrollable infection that existed before the orthopedist was called to see the patient.

The computer attributes an infection to a particular physician because of characteristics of the data system. That is, the physician's name appears in the "attending physician" or "operating surgeon" field. That does not mean that the infection can automatically be attributed to some flaw in the physician's performance.

Figure 9-2

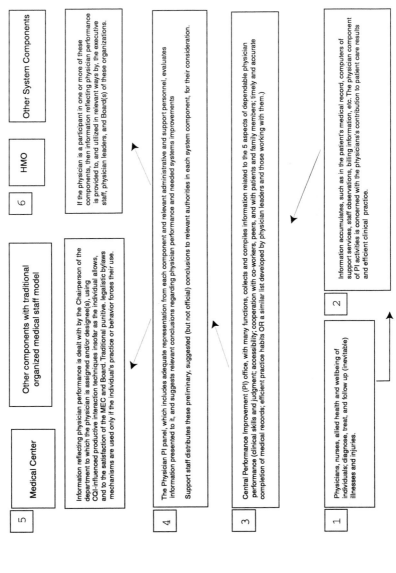

| 5 | Medical Center | | Other components with traditional organized medical staff model | 6 | HMO | | Other System Components |

5 Information reflecting physician performance is dealt with by the Chairperson of the department to which the physician is assigned and/or designee(s), using CQI-influenced productive interaction techniques insofar as the individual allows, and to the satisfaction of the MEC and Board. Traditional punitive, legalistic bylaws mechanisms are used only if the individual's practice or behavior forces their use.

If the physician is a participant in one or more of these components, then information reflecting physician performance is provided to, and utilized in relevant ways by, the executive staff, physician leaders, and Board(s) of these organizations.

4 The Physician PI panel, which includes adequate representation from each component and relevant administrative and support personnel, evaluates information presented to it, and suggests relevant conclusions regarding physician performance and needed systems improvements

Support staff distributes these preliminary, suggested (but not official) conclusions to relevant authorities in each system component, for their consideration.

3 Central Performance Improvement (PI) office, with many functions, collects and compiles information related to the 5 aspects of dependable physician performance (clinical skills and judgment; accessibility; cooperation with co-workers, peers, and with patients and family members; timely and accurate completion of medical records; efficient practice habits OR a similar list developed by physician leaders and those working with them.)

2 Information accumulates, such as in the patient's medical record, computers of support services, staff observations, billing information, etc. The physician component of PI activities is concerned with the physicians's contribution to patient care results and efficient clinical practice.

1 Physicians, nurses, allied health and wellbeing of individuals; diagnose, treat, and follow up (inevitable) illnesses and injuries.

Proper understanding of how to "interpret" clinical information will lead us to develop a "cause-and-effect-adjusted infection rate," if "physician report cards" continue to be considered important. The same is true for mortality rates. Collecting statistics that categorize mortality by face-sheet physician does not equate to eliminating, or confirming, factors that might have contributed to a patient's death.

Statistical Significance vs. Clinical Significance

It is also important to understand that, when the purpose of "analyzing data" is to draw conclusions about the performance of an individual physician, clinical significance overtakes statistical significance at some point. That is, what happens in a few individual cases may be as important as a statistically significant occurrence and "benchmarking."

Example: Let's say a "standard" is established for correct reading of x-rays and imaging studies. Let's make it a high standard, say 90 percent correct readings. Now let's say that a radiologist/imaging specialist meets, indeed exceeds, the standard by being correct 97 times out of 100. It would be misleading to stop there and assume excellent performance. That's because the three cases that were missed may be especially clinically significant (a tumor in the chest behind the heart, a carcinoma of the colon now being treated that is clearly present on earlier studies read as normal, and a tibial plateau fracture of the knee.)

The clinical examples given may be primitive in the reader's eyes, but perhaps they help clarify the point that clinical errors do not have to occur with statistically significant frequency to be of great consequence to patients. Therefore, a system of evaluating physician performance that concerns itself only with statistical significance falls short of achieving the objectives stated on page 63).

8. **Establish a Plan for Smooth Flow of Performance Information.** Figure 9-2 shows one way in which information might flow through an efficient organizational structure. Keys to establishing and maintaining such a system include:

   ‣ Pretend you are the patient. The original intent of using information to confirm physician performance (patient protection) must receive as much attention as any organization-protective components of these activities.

   ‣ Decision-makers in each component of the IHCDS can retain their authority to use results of these activities.

   ‣ The system must be fair to physicians.

   ‣ The system must be as efficient as possible, given the reality of the bureaucratic management layers voluntarily created in some integrated systems.

▸ It is not necessary to duplicate collection of information and committee structures in each component of the IHCDS

▸ Use of information confirming dependable physician perfomance can be component-specific, as long as patient/public interests are well-served.

9. Revisit the "confidentiality" issue. Now that "performance assessment" activities will finally result in the accumulation of positive data confirming good performance, the "confidentiality" issue will disappear, except in situations where an individual's outlier negative performance and/or behavior forces the use of administrative and legal remedies.

Sometimes, to maintain credibility, it may be necessary to share negative information, along with the positive news that continued collection of data shows that efforts to correct the problem have been successful. Change your "confidentiality policy" to a "release of information" policy. In that policy, before you list items of information that are not released without a court order, list all the kinds of positive information you have that you hope people will be interested in seeing.

This transition will be very hard for some traditional-thinking executives, managers and physicians. It may help to recall a basic fact of life:

CONFIDENTIALITY IS A MYTH. SOMEBODY KNOWS.

In the movie "Big Jake," John Wayne plays the part of a tough-guy-family-man whose grandson has been kidnapped. At one point in the movie, Big Jake and his two sons ride boldly into a small town at high noon, with the strongbox of gold to be used for ransom displayed in plain sight. The sons try to dissuade Big Jake from this foolishness, preferring to ride in under cover of darkness, to keep the gold a secret and avoid being robbed. "Nope," says Big Jake. "We're gonna ride right up and show 'em our strength. Never did like secrets. Never knew one that got kept."

Today's successful IHCDSs are discontinuing the foolishness of believing that they can avoid being robbed by hiding the gold. The goal is to ride right up and show the public their strengths. An expected serendipity will be restoration of public and political support for health care managers, executives, and physicians.

References

1. The Atlanta Consulting Group. *America's Healthcare: The Big Squeeze.* La Jolla, Calif.: The Governance Institute, 1996, p. 3.

2. Merry, M. "The Shifting Quality Focus: Implications for Accreditation and Regulation." *The Medical Staff Leadership Forum* (La Jolla, Calif.), Summer 1995, p. 8

3. Thompson, R. *The Medical Staff Leader's Practical Guidebook.* 1st Edition. Marblehead, Mass.: Opus Publications, 1993, pp. 135-48.

4. Accreditation Manuals of the Joint Commission on Accreditation of Hospitals, 1974-1981. Chicago, Ill.: JCAHO.

5. Thompson, R. *The Medical Staff Leader's Practical Guidebook,* 3rd Edition. Marblehead, Mass.: Opus Publications, 1996.

SO YOU'VE BEEN "INTEGRATED": NOW WHAT

PARTICIPATION OF PRACTICING PHYSICIANS IN DECISIONS OF IHCDS MANAGEMENT

Physicians will learn to influence organizational decisions by viewing issues in a broader context than physician self-interest. Paradoxically, physician self-interest will be well-served by this participation.[1]

Increasingly, physicians will _be_ IHCDS management. However, it will still be important for practicing physicians to participate with management in organizational decisions affecting the ability of IHCDS physicians to deliver dependable medical care services.

"Participation" implies a more significant role for practicing physicians than in the days when the operational term was "physician input." "Input" usually meant that physicians could fuss around as much as they wanted to, but they were really at least one step removed from the meeting in which decisions were actually made. In contrast, "participation" implies a meaningful practicing physician voice in decision-making meetings of IHCDS managers, executives, and board members.

This does not mean that practicing physicians should expect the authority to make decisions that are the prerogative of the executive staff and board. Neither should practicing physicians interpret this chapter to mean that each member of the physician panel or medical staff will "have a vote" in the decision. In well-run organizations, there are few general referenda. But practicing physicians are gradually learning that, in terms of influencing organizational decisions (as opposed to political activities), "Who can speak?" is often a much more important question than "Who can vote?" That's because authority (to make the decision), influence, persuasion, and control are not synonyms. Often, a single individual who is an effective persuader can have more influence on and even control over a given situation than a roomful of authorities with lengthy, fancy, official titles.

Figure 10-1. Sample Policy

PARTICIPATION OF PRACTICING PHYSICIANS IN DECISIONS OF RELEVANT IHCDS AUTHORITIES THAT AFFECT THE DELIVERY OF DEPENDABLE MEDICAL CARE SERVICES

To be modified as necessary, then approved by the Governing Boards and Physician Leadership of all components of the IHCDS

This document does not require legal review. It is intended as an organizational guideline, not an absolute legal standard.

Selection of Participating Practicing Physicians

Practicing physicians are selected, ad hoc, to participate in management decisions affecting their areas of clinical practice.

Selection of participating practicing physicians is a joint effort of physician leaders and the relevant IHCDS executive and/or (where applicable) board or management committee.

Practicing physicians selected to participate with management on these occasions will have relevant clinical training and experience, a reputation for objectivity and fairness, good analytical skills, and good communication skills.

Definition of Relevant Authority

Individuals and groups making decisions affecting the delivery of medical services include:

- The system board
- The system CEO
- The board of any system component (if applicable, such as if a hospital or medical center board retains decision-making authority in some areas).
- The CEO, chief operating officer (COO), or vice president in charge of any system component.
- The vice president for medical affairs of the system.
- The vice president for medical affairs or medical director of system components (such as hospital or medical center, mental health services, ambulatory care services, etc.).

Definition of Decisions Affecting the Delivery of Medical Care Services

Decisions affecting delivery of medical care services include, but are not necessarily limited to:

- Planning, construction, and/or renovation of patient care service areas.

Figure 10-1. Continued

- Mergers with or acquisitions of other health care service institutions/organizations in the served area.

- New alliances with physicians in the area served by the system.

- Staffing for various patient care areas, including nurses and other patient care personnel, such as technicians and therapists.

- Selection of practicing physicians, including primary care physicians and the cadre of specialists and subspecialists on whom practicing physicians are dependent for clinical consultation in a variety of circumstances.

- Selection of a clinical support services group, such as pathology or radiology/imaging services.

- Decisions about what services are provided by the various components of the IHCDS.

- Selection of senior executives, as relevant to the activities of practicing physicians.

- Selection of members of the board of directors of the system and members of the board of any system component.

- Funding of education and training programs for clinical personnel including nurses, technicians, and therapists.

- Establishment of reserve funds for capital improvements and contingencies.

Participation Mechanisms

- Specific mechanisms might include, but are not necessarily limited to:

  - Practicing physicians with relevant clinical training and experience on relevant management committees and executive work groups.

  - Physician leaders as full members of relevant board and executive committees.

  - Preparation of fact analyses, position papers, and/or specific recommendations by relevant physician leaders, at the request of the relevant board or management committee or work group.

Participation of practicing physicians (through the implementation of this policy) is reflected in written proceedings, such as minutes and reports, of relevant board and management committees and work groups.

The shift from "physician input" to "physician participation" in organizational decision making is partly due to some trends in organizational leadership. For example, a board is more likely now than in previous years to select a chief executive officer from the growing pool of experienced physician executives. In addition, the participation of a physician executive who is vice president for medical affairs and part of the IHCDS executive staff is more likely to be heeded than the deliberations of a group called a "medical executive committee" that behaves more like a "medical staff legislative committee."

By definition, physician executives are cross-trained in both executive skills and clinical medicine. This balanced senior executive view of factors affecting critical organizational decisions is to the advantage of physicians practicing in the IHCDS and their patients, as well as to the organization itself.

When practicing physicians are offered a chance to participate (even if only with a voice) in organizational decision making, they must be careful not to "blow it." In past years, opportunities for input have justifiably been withdrawn by management if organized groups of aggressive physicians attempted to present "demands" or abused invitations to provide input by using the occasion to scold and intimidate the executive staff and board.

Part of the strategy of living with integration is to learn and practice the two skills necessary to influence management's decisions: (1) objective evaluation and analysis of available information prior to forming an opinion, and (2) carefully prepared, articulate, objective, and calm expression of that opinion to the decision-making group.

Definition of Management Decisions Affecting Patient Care

Perhaps the first insight that articulate practicing physicians provide to management is that it's hard to name a management decision that does not affect the practicing physician's ability to provide dependable medical services. Especially important are decisions involving:

- Planning, construction, and/or renovation of patient care service areas.

- Mergers with or acquisitions of other health care service institutions/organizations in the served area.

- Staffing for various patient care areas, including nurses and other patient care personnel, such as technicians and therapists.

- Choosing practicing physicians whether the mechanism be "credentialing," contracts, or employment.

- Establishment of adequate maintenance and capital improvements funds for clinical service areas.

Methods of Participation

Participation in decision-making meetings has been mentioned. Other methods by which busy practicing physicians can participate in management decision making include telephone conferences and interviews, easy-response questionnaires, and notices to all practicing physicians that they should give their input to the clinical leaders who participate in the decision-making meetings. Note that calling a special meeting is the most ineffective and inefficient method of obtaining clear, relevant, and reliable input from a group of practicing physicians.

Practicing physicians who are most effective in having their input heeded will learn to use whatever input mechanisms are preferred by management. Above all, "physician participation" must never be construed to mean either a demand or an ultimatum, a general vote (31-14 with 3 abstentions), or an expectation that each physician will be asked to express his opinion over lunch with the CEO.

Figure 10-1, pages 72-73, is a sample policy on practicing physician participation in IHCDS management decisions. This sample policy is provided as a template or "menu draft" to be used as a starting point by the team of practicing physician leaders; IHCDS executives, including physician executives; and board members, who together seek to better define "practicing physician participation" in management decisions.

Reference

1. Thompson, R. *Keys to Winning Physician Support.* Tampa, Fla.: American College of Physician Executives, 1991, p. 79.

Chapter 11

THE PRACTICING PHYSICIAN AS EDUCATIONAL RESOURCE FOR THE IHCDS

We need education in the obvious as much as we need investigation of the obscure.[1]

Practicing physicians who like to teach may find it easier to do so as members of an IHCDS professional staff than in the old days of "private practice." That's assuming that practicing physicians in the IHCDS make the effort to convince "management," focused like a horse wearing blinders on this quarter's bottom line, that teaching is an important contribution to the organization's goals of good public image, productivity, and avoidance of legal liability.

Many physicians love both learning and teaching. In fact, as is often pointed out, the word "doctor" comes from the Latin word "docere," meaning "to teach."[2] So, among the practicing physicians in the IHCDS, management can discover a wealth of teaching talent that can be used to good advantage by the organization.

It's routine now for medical centers and IHCDSs to present public general education programs on medical topics such as arthritis, hypertension, and diabetes. This chapter challenges IHCDS management to think also of the value of their practicing physicians as teachers within the organization. Nurses, clinical technicians, and physicians of other specialties enjoy and benefit from continuing education and in-service orientation and training sessions presented by practicing physicians. And sessions in which the realities of clinical practice and clinical decision making are explained to business-trained executives, managers, and lay (nonphysician) board members could do wonders for the legitimacy and practicality of management's decisions.

A major key is for IHCDS management to avoid thinking of time a physician spends teaching as "down time," not directly producing revenue. In fact, in general, it's a brand new concept for many managers trained anytime in the past two decades to understand value in terms other than direct production of revenue. It might help to remind IHCDS management that physicians serve educational needs within the organization without additional pay. And teaching opportunities are part of the reward system for many physicians (see Chapter 4). So opportunities can be counted as a perk rather than as an added "job description" responsibility under "other duties as assigned."

The "bottom line" is that the management of a successful IHCDS will not begrudge time spent by its physicians in educational activities. Au contraire. Insightful IHCDS managers and executives will actively seek opportunities to kill two birds with one stone. That is, take advantage of a valuable educational resource (the practicing physician), while at the same time offering the practicing physician an opportunity to be a teacher.

Such educational activities might include:

- **Part-time clinical faculty assignments at a local Medical University.**"Teaching rounds" with medical students and house staff (residents in training), conducted by practicing physicians, has long been a cornerstone of the fledgling physician's practical education. Today, the IHCDS can reap a large economic benefit from this activity. That is, initial training in medical school must teach the fledgling physician to "do a thorough work-up." That is, leave no stone unturned to arrive at a correct diagnosis. Said another way, order every diagnostic test and imaging study that might possibly pertain to the patient's medical problem.

  Think of the value of having "rounding physicians" who abandon the old, traditional one-upsmanship-game of trying to name a test the medical student has not ordered, but instead frequently ask the medical student, "What did you hope to learn from that test and how did you think getting that test result would affect your plan of care for this patient?" (As the physician reader will recall, the other side of the traditional one-upsmanship-game on "teaching rounds" is for the medical student to cite a relevant recent medical journal article that the rounding physician has not read.)

- **Serving as preceptors.** Preceptorship means that medical students or residents in training, or members of the medical practice community, accompany a practicing physician in the course of his or her daily activities. In the 1980s and early 1990s, legally oriented health care executives feared the legal ramifications of this activity. Today's successful executives work with practicing physicians and full-time medical educators to enhance the public image (therefore the marketability) of the IHCDS by offering such opportunities.

Of course, proper attention should be paid to rules, guidelines, and protocols governing this one-on-one teaching activity, so that the patient is protected from harm and the organization is protected from legal liability. The point is that the old view of a health care executive was most often, "We can't do that because it makes our lawyers nervous." The view of today's successful health care executive is, "We will be aware of and responsive to but not totally constrained by the necessity to safeguard ourselves against legal actions."

- **Providing in-service training and orientation sessions for nurses and clinical technicians.** Traditionally, practicing physicians have been an invaluable resource used by planners of nursing orientation and in-service training sessions, by clinical specialists such as respiratory care technicians and physical therapists, and by support services such as pharmacy and medical records personnel. That is one tradition that should be continued.

- **Providing in-service orientation sessions on clinical topics for members of the executive and management staff who do not have clinical training.** OK, so this one is mostly wishful thinking. The author doesn't really know many senior executive staffs that take advantage of the opportunity to better understand the impact of their decisions by making rounds with practicing physicians.

  But the author (as a patient himself, as well as a taxpayer and former practicing physician) would be delighted if cross-training in the realities of clinical practice were a requirement for all managers and executives presuming to work in the health care field.

- **Speaker's bureau** Physicians have long been popular speakers at civic and community functions. Topics may vary from informing the public about current activities and services available to community members through the IHCDS, to a clinical topic such as, "My Heart Skips Beats: Should I see a Doctor?", to a community-oriented, not self-serving, insight about some current political activity that affects health care.

- **Continuing medical education opportunities.** The IHCDS's medical staff or physician panel will wish to continue the collegial activity of regular continuing medical education sessions at which current journal articles and case studies are discussed and presentations about new clinical advances are made by visiting speakers.
- **Community education.** The presentation of general information

on various medical topics in sessions to which the entire community is invited is one of the most valuable marketing tools an IHCDS can use.

Finally, there is one good parameter by which one can judge the commitment of IHCDS management to education: whether or not the organization believes it is important to fund the establishment, maintenance, and staffing of a good medical library.

References

1. Oliver Wendell Holmes Sr., MD, Professor of Anatomy and Physiology, Harvard University, 1847-1882.

2. *Funk and Wagnall's International Dictionary of the English Language.* Newark, N.J.: Publishers International Press, 1980, p. 374.

Y Chapter 12
YOU AIN'T SEEN NUTHIN' YET

You can always depend on the Americans to do the right thing...after they've tried everything else first.—Winston Churchill

Successful practicing physicians and successful physician executives refuse to get caught up in bandwagon fads. They cut through the maze of acronyms and initialisms, regulations, legalisms, ownership issues, and multilayered organizational structures. Their attention is focused on helping people maintain health as long as possible, then get dependable medical care on the scariest days of their lives.

Thus, practicing physicians and physician executives are properly positioned for the future, no matter what happens next in the world of power politics.

One More Patchwork Fix of the Existing System

Predictably, when the 1996 Congressional and Presidential elections loomed on the horizon, Republican leadership changed its health care policy strategy from obstructionism to action. But legislation touted as "health care reform" does not truly re-form (fundamentally change) the profit-taking system. It only seeks votes by appearing to respond to people's two greatest fears about health care costs and insurance—preexisting condition exclusions and portability of health care coverage from job-to-job. The impact of this policy is certain. Health care insurance premiums will increase.[1]

This political "action" leaves intact a health care system more criticized for its focus on legal and financial maneuvering than it is respected for determining and responding to the needs of the American people. Characteristics of this existing system are summarized in figure 12-1.

Figure 12-1. Existing Health Care Delivery Nonsystem

FEATURE	THE EXISTING HEALTH CARE NONSYSTEM
Coverage	Sporadic
Benefits	Sporadic
Financing (YOU, in one form or another)	Insurance companies, "the government," employers, employees; 60% of health care dollars to hospitals, via "the DRG system."
Special Issues Addressed (LTC, phes, the underinsured, prescription drugs, administrative costs, legal costs, the uninsured)	None (except that, until recently at least, catastro-those with enough money could insure against almost anything)
Cost Control	Utilization management, PRO, certification of need, DRGs, competition (a hodge-podge public policy encouraging profit-taking while ratcheting down revenues; an internal provider bureaucracy that rivals $500 screwdrivers and other waste in the federal bureaucracy)
Physician Payment Plan	Fee for service, RBRVS (resource-based relative value scale); purpose = even out payments, however, the effect was ratcheting down payments to all physicians.
Quality Control	Requirements of the Joint Commission on Accreditation of Healthcare Organizations (JCAHO); "gamed" by providers
Clumping Potential	Positive signs, but motivation of many is to take better advantage of the profit-taking model; acquisitions, takeovers, mergers, short-sighted view of "integrated care" (such as no chiropractic services)
When?	Has grown like Topsy over the past two decades
Where Does My Money Go?	Marketing, consulting and legal fees, high executive compensation, compliance with federal and state regulations, high technology, legal system favors prolonging unproductive life (or at least a heartbeat)

Thompson, R. *Health Care Reform as Social Change*. Tampa, Fla.:
American College of Physician Executives, 1993.

Over the next few years, an anxious public will become increasingly aware of some undesirable features of the managed competition health care model. For example, the profit-taking model invites unwelcome application of antitrust laws to committed efforts to integrate. Also, health care dollars are drained away from paying for needed clinical personnel, space, and equipment to paying instead for trappings of the profit-taking model, such as expensive advertising.

In addition, we cannot hide from the public much longer the degree to which extensive internal layered bureaucracies built voluntarily by providers result in creating more and more top- and mid-level high-paying management positions, instead of emphasizing efficient support for the efforts of clinical practitioners.

Believe it or not, providers at the decision-making level (primarily physicians and executives) will also grow disenchanted with the profit-taking health care model. After the phase of conglomeration, acquisition, and merger, the game will grow less interesting, and less profitable. Investors may lose interest in health care issues as clinical advances reduce the need for revenue-producing, high-tech medical care.

And providers will increasingly appreciate that they are held hostage by the politician/insurer complex. Through masterful political maneuvering on both sides of the aisle, providers find themselves trapped in a mandated health care system that encourages profit-taking with one hand while ratcheting down revenues with the other.

Furthermore, some forward-looking health care executives expert in the financing of mergers and acquisitions, as well as in guiding integrated systems, are shaking their heads in disbelief. At least in private conversation, they are advocates of integrating but appalled by the degree to which conglomeration is occurring. They believe that large conglomerates are leveraging to a dangerous degree and that contingency and capital improvement reserves are inadequate.

As one physician executive (never mind who) wrote this author in response to a letter I wrote and had published in *Physician Executive*,[2] "There will eventually be a collapse of the system and the institution of a single-payer form."

Practicing Physicians: Partners or Pawns?

Forward-looking and knowledgeable executives are also shaking their heads in disbelief as they observe the degree to which physicians are being used as pawns on the gigantic health care chess board.

One author has likened working with physicians to petting a bumblebee.[3] She challenges health care executives to see themselves as "wanting close ties with doctors, but building organizations that won't attract them or hold their interest." She says that it is time to stop "whipping physicians around by one experiment after another" and to begin "building some trust."

Figure 12-2. An Ideal Health Care Delivery System[*]

FEATURE	"IDEAL"
COVERAGE—Covers every citizen of the United States **who cooperates with the rules and pays required premiums and/or taxes**. (This is different from the term "universal," which sends the message, "You live in this country so we owe it to you, whether you contribute or not."	Health care for all ages would be a right of citizenship, as it is now for those over 65 (Medicare) and for certain other groups, such as the handicapped or disabled and dependent children of low-income parents (Medicaid). Call it "universal coverage" if you want, but it's no free handout. The nagging "portability" issue disappears as health care insurance is no longer tied to a single employer. The "insurance industry" as we know it changes in nature, yet people working in the industry are not displaced, as their expertise is critical to implementing the new system. States could be given options in some areas, but some parts of the system (such as quality standards) would be national in scope. Interstate cooperation would be expected/required. Choice of physician is no less than in today's highly touted "managed care" plans. Solves the problem of, "How would managed competition work in rural areas with no or few competitors?
BENEFITS—Encompass all kinds of needed care.	Standard benefits package for all ages, including acute hospital care ("scariest day" care), catastrophic illness, continuous coverage for ambulatory and/or home health care settings, chronic illness (including prescriptions with a reasonable deductible or copayment), and long-term care. Benefits for the disabled and/or handicapped would not be discontinued. "Supplementary" insurance and "long-term care" insurance are rendered obsolete.
FINANCING—**YOU**, in one form or another, in *any* system. The "Medicare Fund" would become the "U.S. Healthcare Fund" and would be enriched by a variety of mechanisms chosen from those explored in the 1993-94 Health Care Reform Debate.	A single payer (the state or federal government, depending on the final details of the plan) would contract with **private-provider-run**, but all not-for-profit, "integrated health care delivery systems" (being developed today, but as profit-making ventures, not service organizations). Competition for a (reasonably) limited number of health care dollars is on the basis of data confirming dependable performance as well as efficient management. Case mix (healthier or sicker) would not be skewed toward one "health care plan" (such as an HMO) or another. Contracts to serve "covered lives" (people in the community) might be given to one provider group for one area of care (such as pediatrics and newborn care), and to another provider group for other areas (such as general medicine and surgery).

84

SO YOU'VE BEEN "INTEGRATED": NOW WHAT

FEATURE	"IDEAL"
FINANCING—YOU Continued	Note that, although there are similarities at first read-ing, this is not a matter of just "picking up" the Canadian system, or the German system, or any other country's system. Neither is it, in the details, the same as either the Clintons' proposals or the Republicans' proposals. And this single-payer, multiple-private-provider plan is not socialized medicine. Socialized medicine is a sin-gle-payer-single-provider system, in which the gov-ernment does everything, with few if any checks and balances. **Properly implemented**, this is a uniquely U.S. system.
SPECIAL ISSUES ADDRESSED	The substantive patient care issues bantered about in the 1993-94 Health Care Reform Debate are addressed (see *Benefits* above). In addition, this plan maintains the competitive mode upon which "man-aged competition" enthusiasts wish to build. But pri-vate providers must compete for a (reasonably) limited number of dollars on the basis of **equal consideration** of data confirming **dependable clinical performance** and efficient financial performance.
PHYSICIAN PAYMENT PLAN	Contract or salary with the IHCDSs . Money would not flow freely to separatist physicians (or separatist hos-pitals). Physicians could choose to opt out of the sys-tem and pursue "private practice," which would be paid for directly by patients/families who also choose to opt out of the system and pay for their own care. Continuous data collection would confirm ongoing dependability of the clinical performance of physicians and physician groups. Methodology to accomplish this task is rapidly developing.
COST CONTROL	Federal or state cost commissions, depending on the final details of the plan, would administer finances. (Any plan can be defeated by enough objection to the idea of trusting the cost and quality commissions. The basic issue in the health care reform debate is trust.) Commission members include leaders of government and business, as well as provider representatives and "public members."

FEATURE	"IDEAL"
QUALITY CONTROL	A National Quality Commission is formed by expanding the Joint Commission on Accreditation of Healthcare Organizations, which already includes "public members" but which is provider-controlled, to include leaders of government and business.
CLUMPING POTENTIAL	Money will not flow to separatists but rather to integrated health care delivery systems, already well on their way to being formed. All such systems would be truly not-for-profit, as opposed to being not-for-profit in name only.
WHEN?	When moderate wings take over both political parties (moderate = problem-solvers, rather than position-takers, who are both fiscally and socially responsible) or when a truly independent President is elected to work with a Congress with a majority of Independent members.
MEDICARE CONTINUES?	No, but currently existing Medicare funds are used to begin support of the new program, under which additional funds become available for **all** age groups, including those over 65.
WHERE DOES MY MONEY GO?	Money goes to pay for health care services, rather than for trappings of the profit-taking model such as advertising and investor profit. But this won't happen automatically. There must be guidelines, and **there must be accountability**.

* *Between the Lines* (The TMA Press, Dunedin, Fla.) 1(5):5-6, Nov.-Dec. 1995.

Other authors have pointed out that decision-makers, such as executives and board members, must put aside the past paradigm of "obtaining physician input" and proceed to true partnership participation by grass-roots practicing physicians as well as by entrepreneurial and organizational physician leaders.[4,5,6]

Life after Managed Competition

Over time, a new provider/public coalition will emerge that will be powerful enough to influence the politician/insurer complex. Development of that powerful new coalition awaits only the realization that providers and the public are not enemies. The interests of providers and the public may not be totally the same, but they are at least inextricably intertwined.

Through both political action and substantive activities in integrated settings, the U.S. health care system will gradually develop characteristics similar to those depicted in figure 12-2. The public will insist that a central place in this system be occupied by practicing physicians and physician executives who have gained experience in today's evolving integrated health care delivery systems.

Forging the Future

The future can be anticipated in two ways. Some sit in front of their television sets to be told what the future holds; then they react. Others are like the baseball umpire who was asked, "How do you tell a strike from a ball?" "Easy," replied the umpire, "considering that it ain't either one 'til I call it."

Six lessons learned from the Great Health Care Reform Debate of 1993-94 can help practicing physicians forge the future rather than be controlled by the future:

1.   The biggest issue in health care is not money; it is trust. Practicing physicians hold a trump card in the trust of their patients, who are thankful for good medical care.

2.   Lack of trust in the system is too often justified. The relationship between economic value and respect for human values is too often lost when the overriding objective is to exploit people in need of medical care services to maximize investor profit.

3.   The existing political alignment is wrong. Manipulation by politicians and insurers, carelessness and perceived indifference by providers, and ambitious investigative reporters have caused the public to lose trust in the commitment of health care practitioners

and organizational leaders. The winning strategy of today's successful integrated system is to build a provider/public coalition powerful enough to deal effectively with the politician/insurer complex.

4. Information confirming dependable performance must be developed, interpreted, and shared. An information-oriented public must be given data to confirm that providers are not increasing profit by cutting corners that make medical care services less dependable. In addition, members or beneficiaries of health care plans must be provided data-based assurance of the dependable performance of individual physicians.

5. "Profit taking" and "competition" are not synonyms. Competition will exist in a uniquely U.S. health care system with some features borrowed from the single-payer model and some features borrowed from the market-forces model, regulated by a combination of state and federal rules. (See figure 12-2).

6. Money will not flow easily to separatists, whether a freestanding physician practice, a freestanding hospital, or even a freestanding system. Success depends on reasonable integration of medical care services.

Six Action Guidelines

These insights suggest six action guidelines for the practicing physician/physician executive team:

1. **Continue efforts to integrate**. This includes persuading state and federal legislators that application of antitrust laws must not be allowed to defeat well-meaning efforts to avoid needless duplication of services.

2. **Encourage responsible decision making**. Attorneys will be the true decision makers in health care until physicians and other leaders in the integrated system break the habit of asking attorneys to make decisions that they should make themselves.

   In a discussion session, such as for a few minutes prior to a business meeting or during a weekend retreat, create four lists:
   - Five good reasons to ask an attorney for information (then make our own decision).
   - Five times we don't need an attorney after all.
   - Five good reasons to ask a consultant for help.
   - Five times we don't need a consultant after all.

3. **Be effective public educators.** Build the provider/public coalition.

4. **Define "quality" as "dependable performance."** Stop claiming that "quality" is an ephemeral, ethereal, elusive concept chased after only by academic philosophers. Define "quality" as "dependable performance" from the viewpoint of users of medical care services.

5. **Revisit "confidentiality."** When trust is a major issue, those who hide data invite the suspicion that there must be something to hide.

6. **Reexamine the concept of "value."** Rediscover the relationship between economic value and personal values. Personal values of physicians, executives, and board members determine the relative priorities assigned to profit on one hand and service on the other. And properly balancing those two concerns is a critical key to success in any business.

The Surest Prediction of All

The most significant "health care reform" in U.S. history was led by practicing physicians right after World War I. (President Woodrow Wilson's political attempts to reform the U.S. health care system had been defeated by the insurance industry and by the fact that he had proposed a model much like the one Bismarck had established in Germany.) The focus of those early reformers was not cost. It was patient care. The vehicles of that reform were the Flexner report on the status of U.S. medical education and the Standard for Hospitals promulgated by the American College of Surgeons.[7]

Now, history is about to repeat itself. Politicians have had their chance, and they have failed. Recent changes driven by executives trained only in finance and business management have only reflected an overzealous interpretation of competition and focused on the goal of maximizing investor profit.

Now up to bat are teams of practicing physicians and physician executives who truly understand the fundamental nature and functions of a successful, dependable integrated health care delivery system.

References

1. Wallsten, P. "Insurer to Raise Its Rates in July." *St. Petersburg Times*, June 8, 1993, p. E1.

2. Thompson, R. "Reader Feedback." *Physician Executive* 22(3):46-7, March 1996.

3. Grayson, M. "How To Pet a Bumblebee." *Hospitals & Health Networks* 70(3):7, Feb. 5, 1996.

4. Goldsmith, J. "Driving the Nitroglycerin Truck." *Healthcare Forum Journal* 36(3):35-44, March/April 1993.

5. Thompson, R. *Keys to Winning Physician Support.* Tampa, Fla.: American College of Physician Executives, 1991.

6. Sandrick, K. "How to Succeed with Doctors by Really Trying." *Hospitals & Healthcare Networks* 70(3):23-8, Feb. 5, 1996.

7. *The Minimum Standard for Hospitals.* Chicago, Ill.: American College of Surgeons, 1919.

GLOSSARY

Several jargon words and phrases are being used by a lot of different individuals and groups to mean a lot of different things. Here's a list of some terms used in this book and what they mean, in the context of this book.

Administrator is used in the neutral, dictionary sense of "one who administers something," such as logistical details related to buildings, budgets, planning, personnel, and needs of people in an organization. See also *health care manager*.

Clinical Practice does not mean "private practice" or any other practice arrangement. It means the difficult task of modifying *clinical pathways* and *practice guidelines* to fit the unique needs of each person receiving *medical care services* in the various clinical settings that are components of the *IHCDS*.

Clinical Pathways are step-by-step roadmaps for the care of specific medical problems. They include activities of all clinical professionals (practicing physicians, nurses, clinical technicians) on whom a patient depends for *medical care services*.

Health Care is a term used by politicians, insurance companies, and managers of provider organizations to encompass all types of *medical care services* provided by *IHCDSs*.

Health Care Executive is a term preferred by senior managers in *IHCDSs* and their components.

Health Care Manager means an individual providing needed support to physicians, nurses, and clinical technicians delivering *medical care services*.

IHCDS means Integrated Health Care Delivery System. IHCDS is not synonymous with *managed care* system, HMO, PHO, or any other jargon term implying a health care policy of allowing market forces to control costs and ensure dependability of *medical care services*. Rather, IHCDS simply means an opportunity for people in need of any medical care service to receive it from the same provider. An IHCDS is true reality, an entity that can be visited. In an IHCDS, physicians, nurses, and clinical technicians work with people (patients, residents, clients, and family members) supported by management. The focus is on meeting the needs of people in need of either preventive or therapeutic medical care services.

Managed Care, in this book, is reserved to mean management of the individual patient (or client or resident, whatever is applicable in the various components of the *IHCDS*) by clinical practitioners who modify *clinical pathways* and *practice guidelines* to fit the unique needs of members and beneficiaries who are users of *medical care services* offered by the *IHCDS.*

Managed Competition describes the current U.S. health care system, unique in the world because the goal of the system is investor profit.

Medical Care Services, in this book, means the spectrum of services delivered by a physician/nurse/clinical technician team to inpatients, outpatients, residents, or clients (as applicable) in the various components of an *IHCDS*, which include settings concerned with maintenance of physical, mental, and emotional health.

This usage is adopted in this book because the distinction between "health care services" and "medical care services" is an artificial one, and use of the term "health care services" promotes divisiveness between practicing physicians and other clinical professionals and managers when what is needed is cooperative effort.

Also, while politicians, policy-makers, and *IHCDS* management may be concerned with broad aspects of "health care," the public is primarily concerned with the dependability of specific *medical care services* provided to individual patients and families.

Organization means an entity that exists only on paper. An organization is virtual reality, as opposed to true reality (see *IHCDS*).

Practice Guidelines differ from *clinical pathways* in that they specifically relate to the clinical decision-making process of the practicing physician, who is the CEO in the context of caring for individual patients. Tailoring of practice guidelines to match the unique characteristics of individual patients and the specific manifestations of their medical problems (*see clinical practice*) sets the *IHCDS's* systems in motion and modifies *clinical pathways* that involve activities of clinical practitioners in addition to physicians.

Practicing Physician means an MD or DO whose primary activity is providing the physician component of *medical care services* provided to members or beneficiaries of the *IHCDS*. See *clinical practice.*

Quality, in the context of this book, means dependable performance from the viewpoint of users of *medical care services* provided by an *IHCDS*

EPILOGUE

Pretend You Are the Patient

It's November 25, 2005. Happy Golden Anniversary to us. At age 70, Joan and I are among the lucky ones. We are sheltered safely in our large home complete with pool and Drexel Heritage furniture, secure in the love of family and a good return on our investments.

Totally secure. Except for two uncertain factors that we cannot control, and therefore try not to think about. One factor is when (not whether, but when) our big scary day will come, which of us will be first, and whether the scare will be cancer or a heart attack. The other uncertain factor is related to the first. We cannot control the hour and cause of our death. (But the recently passed Federal Euthanasia Act is on the President's desk awaiting signature or veto.)

Listen outside. My hearing is not what it used to be. Is that a siren? No? Well, maybe not right here, not right now. But all across America, in towns large and small, hundreds of blaring sirens broadcast the urgency of emergency vehicles racing against time, carrying people whose scary days have come. The people in the ambulances are no longer just U.S. citizens. Tonight they are, through no choice of their own, patients plus concerned family members. They did their best to comply with the state's Fitness and Wellness Program mandates. But they could not avoid the fact that the death rate in the United States has not declined. The U.S. death rate is one apiece. No waiver for physicians.

So someday, like the people in the ambulances, Joan and I will be dependent on the health care system we have helped to build. And so will our children. And so will our grandchildren. And so will you. And so will your children. And so will your grandchildren.

Meanwhile, our security is a restless security. And so is yours. Even though you are a physician, there will always be two uncertain factors threatening your security which you cannot control...except insofar as you pretend you are the patient as you build today's and tomorrow's integrated health care delivery systems.